T0113364

The Virility
Solution

*Everything You Need to Know About
Viagra, the Potency Pill That Can Restore and
Enhance Male Sexuality*

Steven Lamm, M.D.
and Gerald Secor Couzens

A FIRESIDE BOOK
Published by Simon & Schuster

FIRESIDE
Rockefeller Center
1230 Avenue of the Americas
New York, NY 10020

First Fireside Edition 1999

FIRESIDE and colophon are registered trademarks
of Simon & Schuster Inc.

Designed by Irving Perkins Associates, Inc.
Line illustrations by Tim Jeffs
Manufactured in the United States of America

1   3   5   7   9   10   8   6   4   2

Library of Congress Cataloging-in-Publication Data
Lamm, Steven.
The virility solution / Steven Lamm and Gerald Secor Couzens.
p.   cm.
1. Sildenafil.   2. Phentolamine.   3. Impotence—Chemotherapy.
I. Couzens, Gerald Secor.   II. Title.
RC889.L28   1998
616.6'92061—dc21   98-5837
CIP
ISBN 0-684-84780-9
0-684-85431-7 (Pbk)

The International Index of Erectile Function (IIEF) Questionnaire, by Raymond C.
Rosen, Alan Riley, Gorm Wagner, Ian Osterloh, John Kirkpatrick, and Avanish Mishra,
from *Urology*, vol. 49 (6), 1997, 822–30, is reprinted with the permission of
Elsevier Science.

To Kiki, wife, friend, confidant, and lover. To my parents, the late Dr. Arnold Lamm and Lucy, who continues to give me so much love. To my special Yvonne. And to the children, David, Suzanne, Alexandra, Owen and Morgan.

S.L.

To Elisa, Gerald, Dominic, Mary, and Rose, all of my love. And to Frank X. Michel, who has helped me more than I can ever say.

G.S.C.

Contents

A Word from the Author

What a remarkable year it's been! In the months following the release of Viagra and the publication of the hardcover edition of *The Virility Solution,* millions of prescriptions have been written in the United States, shattering all records for a new drug. The same popular trend has subsequently occurred in scores of other countries around the globe where Viagra has been approved for use. Like other medications that have quickly gone from use by thousands, in closely controlled scientific studies, to millions with all types of medical backgrounds, it's not unusual for some serious side effects to be noted. While fatal heart attacks have initially been linked to Viagra use, a closer look at the medical evidence reveals other causes for death, not only Viagra-related but also linked to serious underlying medical conditions. According to the Food and Drug Administration, Viagra is still an extremely safe medication when properly prescribed.

Just as deaths due to heart attacks brought on by physical activities such as jogging or shoveling snow have been well documented in the medical literature, deaths from heart attacks during sexual activity have also been noted. Heart attacks are typically caused by complex factors that affect the blood's coagulation system. We are aware of many heart attack triggers—but not all of them.

Recent research points out that the odds of having a heart attack after having sex are about 2 per million for a healthy fifty-year-old man. For a man who has had a previous heart attack, the odds are higher, but still minuscule: 20 per million. Clearly, the older the man, the higher the risk of heart attack during and after sexual activity. It goes without saying that being in excellent physical condition improves your odds considerably. Those men with heart disease who exercise three or more times a week will have a significant reduction in their risk of heart attack. On the other hand, the sedentary, unfit person with heart disease has increased his risk threefold of suffering a heart attack during and after sex.

Unfortunately, in addition to being a very serious health matter, heart disease is all too common. Each year, more than 500,000 people in the U.S.

7

survive a heart attack; more than 10 percent of the population is living with heart disease. Some of my patients between the ages of forty and fifty have already suffered their first heart attacks. Even so, heart disease doesn't mean that sexual intimacy has to come to an end. Before prescribing Viagra for some of my cardiac patients, I have them first submit to a special "Viagra Stress Test" I've devised that's conducted for me by a local cardiologist.

Here's how the Viagra Stress Test works. One hour after a 50 mg dose of Viagra is taken, the man is then put through a standard cardiac stress test, which is taken by either jogging on a treadmill or by pedaling an exercise bike. Under the supervision of the cardiologist, the physical resistance is increased incrementally over a period of minutes, making the man's heart pump harder to keep up with the exertion—just as it would during sexual activity. Blood pressure and electrocardiogram readings are taken regularly to assess the man's stamina and health as the physical task becomes harder. When testing is finally completed and the man is given the green light from the cardiologist, I will then write a Viagra prescription for him with great assurance, knowing that sexual activity coupled with Viagra will not be hazardous to his health.

It's now well known that commonly prescribed nitrate-based heart medications cannot be used if Viagra is to be prescribed. Of the dozens of men who have died worldwide after taking the diamond-shaped blue pill, many were taking nitrates, a medication that Pfizer, the manufacturer of Viagra, has clearly warned may cause a deadly drop in blood pressure. Other men had underlying medical conditions, along with problems with blood pressure, which also explained their predisposition to heart attack after sexual intercourse.

As time goes on, doctor and patient alike should be aware that as millions more men begin to take Viagra, we will come to learn about other prescription medications that may result in a negative interaction with Viagra. Medications that lower blood pressure, used in conjunction with Viagra, may result in an exaggerated response by lowering blood pressure excessively in some patients. Currently, several medications have been found to increase the rate at which Viagra is metabolized by the body, possibly affecting the ability to have a satisfactory erection: cimetidine (Tagamet), erythromycin, and ketoconazole (Nizoral). The drugs itraconazole (Sporanox) and rifampin have been found to have just the opposite effect, actually delaying the effect of Viagra when taken concurrently. The FDA is constantly monitoring the use of Viagra, its drug–drug interactions, and continually updates physicians and the public about what adjustments need to be made.

With the incredible success and popularity of many of our prescription medications, it should not be forgotten that each one still carries a potential risk, which is why medications have to be prescribed by a physician who will detail all possible interactions and side effects. For the most recent updates regarding Viagra, or any of the newer erectile agents, you may go to my Internet Web site: www.virilitysolution.com.

The Medical Miracle That Can Change Your Life

FINALLY, IT'S FRIDAY, Dennis thought to himself as he made the turn off the freeway toward his house in Silicon Valley. Exhausted, with another sixty-hour workweek behind him, he looked forward to some well-deserved rest and relaxation at home. There, he knew Jennifer would be waiting for him with a bottle of chilled white wine, the stereo playing softly in the background, and the big leather sofa waiting to envelop them.

When he opened the front door he was already anticipating the evening ahead. It didn't matter that his body and mind were tired enough for ten hours of sleep; he'd be otherwise engaged, soon. Greeting Jennifer with a kiss, he settled himself down in the living room, and waited for her to join him.

Very soon she did, carrying a tray with a bottle of wine, two glasses, and a small china plate with a small blue pill for Dennis. Both he and Jennifer knew that it would ensure them a night of intense sexual pleasure, and the anticipation of those events brought a flush to both their faces. With that pill, their weekend, their sex lives, and most of all their ongoing relationship would be enhanced and enriched.

Jennifer poured the wine and passed Dennis a glass. He leaned over, picked up the pill, and, toasting his wife, swallowed it. Both Jennifer and Dennis were willing participants in the new world of sexual medicine, which gave them the security of knowing that they could have what they wanted, when they wanted it.

Everyone can.

All adults are entitled to a fulfilling sex life. An active component of complete health, the ability to have satisfying sex is a marker signifying that all the elements which define us are working together seamlessly. By this I mean not only the physical, but the very important psychological and emotional factors as well. What it comes down to is this: sex is good for you.

As an internist in New York City, I see patients who represent a cross section of the population, from every background and of every age. They come to me for a range of reasons, from yearly checkups to follow-ups to surgery, and everything in between. Increasingly, however, my male patients are coming in to discuss their sex lives and, more specifically, their inability to consistently have erections. Whether they are in their thirties, forties, fifties, sixties, or older, this vital part of their being can sometimes falter, for any number of reasons. Wanting to be the best they can be, at every stage of their lives, they ask about the options available to them.

My goal is to give them the best that medical science has to offer to help restore erections. Today, there are extraordinary new additions to the world of prescription medicine which, without a doubt, rank among the most exciting discoveries in recent medical research. Drugs which accomplish what millions of men, and their partners, have been waiting for are finally available.

For every man who is worried about the possible loss of potency —the ability to have a firm erection each and every time he wants to have sex—for every male who has already experienced it, and for every partner who ever wondered what to do, there is not only hope, there is this new medical miracle.

Simply stated, a revolution has begun. Most men who suffer from erectile dysfunction, or ED, may now restore their virility by taking a prescription pill. The impact on the estimated thirty million men who experience ED cannot be underestimated. *Today, ED can be treated successfully more than 95 percent of the time. Nevertheless, fewer than 5 percent of those affected have received treatment.*

Effective, and well tolerated, these amazing pharmacological virility remedies are Viagra, the brand name for sildenafil, and Vasomax (phentolamine). For the first time, it is possible to restore optimal sexual function to nearly every man who desires it. *And they will put to rest the myth that ED is an irreversible function of aging.* In a matter of minutes, the new oral medications can:

- allow a man to have firmer erections to ensure fulfilling sexual intercourse
- renew and strengthen an existing—or even dormant—sex life
- bolster self-confidence
- lift depression associated with ED, thereby positively affecting all facets of a man's life, including his work
- help to create a relaxed, unhurried window of opportunity to proceed at a couple's individual pace
- mend relationships torn by frustration
- offer joy in the sexual arena, where little or none had been felt for years
- solidify sexual bonds with a partner
- restore intimacy and thereby deepen relationships

THE RELATIONSHIP PILLS

My growing awareness of the great need for such a medical intervention was sparked by my patients, as is often the case. In their visits to me, most bring with them their hopes and fears as well as colds and worries about cholesterol counts. This was the case with Mark and his wife, Lucy.

Mark, a thirty-eight-year-old bond trader on Wall Street, was certainly healthy. A handsome man with movie-star good looks, he had been coming to see me for five years, but in this visit something in his demeanor seemed to have changed. I asked him point-blank if anything in particular was bothering him.

"There's a lot of stress in my life—more than usual," he told me. "With the type of economy we've got going, I see no end to the stress. It's make-or-break time for me and my partners."

"How is that affecting your eating and sleeping patterns?" I asked. "And what about your quality of life in general?"

"I'm pretty good about what I eat," he said, avoiding the last question. "But I could be sleeping better. And, I have to confess, I'm drinking more wine with dinner. I really need it to decompress."

Since all of Mark's tests were in the normal range and I didn't suspect anything physically amiss, I suggested that he limit himself to one glass of wine a night and try to get an extra hour of sleep. As he was preparing to leave, I inquired after Lucy.

"She's great," he said brusquely and hurried out the door.

It so happened that Lucy's yearly appointment was the following week. She, too, checked out fine physically, but seemed subdued and anxious. I knew something had changed since I last saw her, and I wondered what it was. Obviously it was affecting both husband and wife.

"Did Mark speak to you?" she asked.

Not certain what she was referring to, I shook my head no.

"He promised he would," she said with a sigh.

Gently, I asked her what was bothering her.

"It's not just me—it's both of us," she said. "But it's not right for me to speak to you alone. I'm going to talk to him tonight and try to convince him that we both should see you—together."

Whatever Lucy said to Mark after leaving my office clearly had the desired effect. A couple of weeks later the two of them came to see me, looking rather tense and nervous.

"I know something is wrong and I want to help you both," I said. "But without knowing what the problem is, I'm stuck."

"Okay," Mark began. "Here it is. Our sex life has not been working right for the last ten months—because *I'm* not working right. I can't get a hard-on. I thought it was the stress and the alcohol. I actually stopped drinking altogether after my checkup—I read somewhere that alcohol can affect performance—but it hasn't helped. Not only is my personal life suffering, so is my professional one. Frankly, it's a bummer. My confidence is shaken," he admitted.

"You're right about drinking," I agreed. "It can often inhibit penile function."

"But if that's not the cause, and there isn't something physically wrong with Mark, then maybe *I'm* doing something wrong," Lucy said. "We have a strong relationship in every way and we don't believe we need marriage counseling, but maybe we will if we can't get back on track sexually. What can we do?"

The solution, I told them, might just be ready and waiting for them. "Your experience is a very common one, more usual than most people think," I said. "Mark, given the results of your recent checkup, I have no reason to believe that your erection problems have a physical cause. They are probably due to your increased business pressure. I call it the 'phenomenon of busy people' and I'm seeing it in more and more of my patients.

"Hopefully, there will be a time when the pressure eases up and you can resume a more relaxed workweek. Maybe that will help your erections. In the meantime, however, there is an effective solution. There are two new safe medications in pill form that help restore erections, no matter what the primary cause of the problem is. One of the drugs, Vasomax, is what I have been using with men as part of an ongoing study for a pharmaceutical company. The other, Viagra, is also undergoing review, but in other centers around the United States. I'm still enrolling patients and their partners. And since you are both here, would you like to join the trial?"

I explained that the best aspect of these medications is the unique way in which they react biochemically as facilitators and amplifiers of erections. But there must be normal sexual stimulation in order for an erection to occur. In other words, emotion and caring play a big part in how they work successfully. But one thing is certain: they will help a man achieve the best possible combination of desire and physical functioning.

Their expressions mirrored their skepticism, but Mark and Lucy were ready to try anything. After Mark and Lucy signed the necessary papers required for the study and I took a blood sample, I gave him a Vasomax pill to swallow. I noted his blood pressure and heart rate over the course of the next hour. A possible side effect of Vasomax is a sharp decrease in blood pressure and an associated rise in pulse. If his blood pressure dropped by more than 30 points over his predose reading, Mark would be ineligible to use the drug. His blood pressure dropped only 10 points, with no other noticeable change to him. His pulse went up 10 beats per minute, which was to be expected. Mark was eligible for the trial and I supplied him with a month's worth of the drug.

Several days later, I received a fax from Mark with just two words: "It worked!"

And a few months later, Mark was not only his old self, he was even better. He was surprised to find that on some occasions he no longer required the medication to achieve an erection. His job perfor-mance was stronger than before and he was drinking moderately, if at all. Most importantly, he understood how his ED had developed and hoped that soon he would not need the medication at all. But should his ED recur—for whatever reason—he felt confident knowing that he could go back on the medication under my supervision.

The Intergenerational Drugs

Mark was so impressed with the results of taking Vasomax that he convinced his father to pay me a visit. A widower for four years, Jim, at sixty-five, had recently met a woman whom he felt at home with and who made him laugh. While he never thought he would be sexually attracted to another woman again, to his amazement he now was. Unfortunately, the new pair's budding sex life was at a standstill because Jim couldn't get an erection. He was worried that Emily, at fifty-four, would give up on him.

The first thing I did, as I always do with a new patient, was take a medical history. Then I had a lengthy conversation with Jim on his habits and any changes he noticed in himself.

"I'm not really comfortable carrying around the extra twenty-five pounds I've gained in the last couple of years," he admitted. "But what really troubles me is my inability to have sex. I can only get about as hard as a limp noodle and it makes me feel terrible. After my wife died, I was depressed for a long time. Then I met Emily and started to feel sexual desires and longing for a woman once again. And now this—"

I explained to Jim that ED is sometimes a sign of illness and I wanted to give him a checkup to rule out that possibility. After a thorough examination, it turned out that, unlike his son, Jim's ED was not brought on by lifestyle factors. The true culprit was an undiagnosed case of diabetes.

STEVEN LAMM, M.D.

"Type II diabetes, the kind you have, is very common," I explained. "It can start as early as age thirty, although it's much more usual in middle age, and the majority of those with the disease are often over-weight."

"But I don't feel sick," Jim replied.

"The symptoms of type II diabetes are slow to appear," I told him. "ED is often the first real sign that something is wrong. In fact, about half of all the men in whom diabetes has been detected will develop some form of ED within ten years of the onset of the disease."

"So how does diabetes put the brakes on my sex life?"

"For the most part, the ED is induced by vascular disease caused by the diabetes, which results in blood vessel blockages, including the arteries of the penis. Nerves can also be damaged by the disease, which is another factor that hurts your erection capabilities."

"So, can you fix my problems?" he asked hopefully.

"First of all, control of your diabetes is your most critical health issue right now," I said. "That means you must make a serious effort to lose the extra weight you have put on over the last few years. And you can do that through regular exercise and adjustments in your diet. As for your erection problem, I can tell you this: while your specific type of ED is *not* curable, because it's caused by diabetes, which is a chronic disease, it may be able to be successfully treated with a new oral medi-cation."

I explained to Jim that in the future Viagra would be one of the new medications available to him and that it had a great likelihood of being effective despite the strong biological impact of diabetes on his erectile performance. At the present time, I was using Vasomax in my study. Although it is less effective for men with moderate to severe dysfunction, it can work well for those with either mild to moderate dysfunction or ED caused by psychological reasons.

I told Jim it was certainly worth trying Vasomax because it was well tolerated, with an excellent safety profile. I explained how the

16

Vasomax study worked and offered him the opportunity to enroll as long as he met all the criteria. He did and three weeks later he called me. "I'm a private kind of guy, but I just had to tell you what happened," he told me. "It's been great, being able to really feel again and give Emily pleasure. It just made us grow even closer. I'm a complete man again. I can't thank you enough. It's a miracle—and I never thought I'd live to see it."

Jim's response gave me two reasons to be thrilled. One, I knew that the quality of Jim's life had improved. And, two, the fact that he had responded to Vasomax pointed out that his diabetes was not as advanced as I had feared. Jim has since shed the extra weight, his diabetes is under control with Glyburide, an oral diabetes treatment, and he still takes his ED medication. The beauty of both Viagra and Vasomax is that they are compatible with drugs most commonly prescribed by physicians.

THE PSYCHOLOGICAL LINK

Psychological causes of ED are not unusual. In fact, it's estimated that up to 50 percent of all cases fall into this category. Given the times we live in, and the way the roles of men and women have changed in the last twenty years, in addition to the expectations we hold ourselves to, 5o percent isn't surprising.

Take the case of Robert and Jane. Their six-year marriage had hit serious snags and they were working—seemingly to no avail—with a psychiatrist to iron things out. Robert had trouble getting an erection, and seven months of very expensive therapy was fueling his anger, making his ED a burden that grew heavier day after day.

The primary conflict in their marriage was Jane's career. While Robert was proud of her accomplishments—she was a successful and highly visible banker—he chafed at her absences from home. And although he certainly admired her financial acumen and respected her choice to keep her personal finances and investments separate from his, the fact that she was more savvy at it than he was bothering him.

Jane, on her part, craved intimacy with her husband. She knew that her extended absences were a strain on their marriage and she felt that closeness was even more important those times when she was home. But when she was there, she was tired and sex wasn't necessarily what she needed or wanted.

Robert, on the other hand, began to feel that Jane's frequent absences were growing proof that she didn't really love him. And when they did have time for sex, he found, to his growing dismay, that he was often unable to achieve an erection. His anxiety increased, leading to more erectile failure, which, in turn, led to even more worry about his performance in bed. Eventually, he avoided any kind of physical closeness altogether.

Jane took his behavior as a clear sign that he was no longer interested in her. One night, they finally had the confrontation that had been building for months. When Robert, after two glasses of Scotch, told Jane that her career left no room for him and made him feel worthless, she was stunned. The ultimate accusation was even worse: his ED, he said, was her fault.

Stung by his words, Jane knew they were at a turning point in their marriage. Fortunately, she had heard about the clinical trials of the new oral ED medications from a colleague. Feeling there was nothing to lose, she mentioned them and offered to accompany Robert to my office.

Because he initially felt that his wife was taking charge of yet another facet of their lives, Robert took a couple of days to think it over. Then he made the decision to see me. And for both of them, their marriage did turn—but this time, they found the footing they needed to head in the right direction. Acknowledging that she had to make changes, too, Jane cut back on her travel and began to spend more time with her husband. Robert responded to the erection pills; his anger and anxiety diminished and his self-confidence returned.

Now they began to make headway in their work with the psychiatrist, and they were willing and able to address the issues that concerned them. Defining what intimacy and sex meant to each of them, as well as dealing with the problems brought about by careers and finances, brought them closer. And as their communication skills improved, their relationship flourished. Over time, Robert's erectile difficulties began to vanish. Soon, he found that he didn't always need a pill to achieve an erection.

But the best part of this story is this: the effect of psychotherapy is jump-started by the medication, and the time an ED patient will spend in a therapist's office is, therefore, vastly reduced. Had Robert come to me for the medication as soon as his problem began, I might have been able to shorten his time on the psychiatrist's couch by half.

Mark, Jim, and Robert are just three of my many patients who have had their sex lives fully restored using the new medications. Whether the syndrome is provoked by changes in circumstances, which cause a temporary and easily rectified problem, or by ongoing worries about endurance, past performance, or other conditions, this medication regimen can help. Its effect is so profound that it is capable of aiding those men who suffer from ED as the result of certain diseases. It can even produce startling results for men who have suffered with ED for a decade or more.

THE RATIONAL TREATMENT

The search for a safe, painless, and efficient solution to ED has been a long and arduous one. Many physicians, myself included, as well as the patients we've treated, have been dissatisfied with the old medical options—none of which included a pill. Previously, the only choices for men were injections into the shaft of the penis, a vacuum device to increase rigidity, or the insertion of bendable rods into the penis. None of these past interventions, two of which were physically invasive, was totally satisfactory.

Today, sexual medicine is in its infancy and virility programs are just beginning to come into use. Viagra has only recently been approved for general use by the Food and Drug Administration (FDA), with FDA approval of Vasomax expected shortly. So it's understandable that many millions of men are unaware of the new oral medications that are at their physician's disposal. With such medications, their erectile problems can be treated immediately, successfully, and unobtrusively.

Beginning in 1997, I had the opportunity to work, with my medical colleagues, in the testing of Vasomax for the treatment of ED. Both Vasomax and Viagra had been in use for several years in worldwide medically supervised programs and the results had been nothing less than astounding. These two miraculous pharmaceuticals temporarily correct ED in a natural manner. This is because they require an appropriate sexually stimulating environment in order for an erection to occur. These drugs do not increase sexual desire. What they do so well is enhance performance that grows out of sexual desire. If a man takes either pill and is not physically attracted to his partner, he is not going to get results. That's what makes these drugs so revolutionary: for the first time since birth control pills were prescribed, the effects of a drug touch the sex lives of two people: the one who takes it *and* his partner.

While the previous methods of enhancing an erection were effective, they worked in a very rudimentary fashion. None of them required a partner. Neither stimulation nor the desire of a partner was needed in order for these sex aids to bring on an erection. For this major reason, many women found themselves excluded from the process. This has all changed with the erection pill. All it takes is a prescription from your doctor.

You Can Take Control

ED is an unbiased condition. It affects men of all ages and circumstances, whatever their sexual habits or preferences. At least one out of every three men over the age of fifty will experience it. Men whose sex lives are irregular, due to any number of causes, can suffer from ED to the same extent as men with more frequent sexual encounters. But ED is not about standards of performance or an arbitrary scale of how frequently you should or need to have sex. After all, our sex lives are private and dependent on the two people involved. But whatever causes the problem, it can now be treated quickly and painlessly.

For decades, ED was believed to be a psychological rather than a physiological problem. However, in many cases, the problem is physical or oftentimes a combination of both. And, like other medical conditions, it may require medication. Do you believe that high blood pressure is a "mental" problem? Or that your cholesterol level is based on what's "in your head"? Or, even worse, that if a medical problem is left untreated, it will just go away? I sincerely hope not.

Modern medicine has treatments for many of today's ailments, and now an incredibly effective medication has been added to its arsenal. However, as with any complaint, your doctor can't treat you unless you tell him, or her, what is wrong. As both a man and a physician, I understand that there is probably no other medical condition which has so great a potential to frustrate, humiliate, and devastate as ED. You may have been too embarrassed to mention the problem or you may have gone to your doctor in the past and been given choices that were so off-putting and emotionally punishing that you chose to forgo help. I myself was always displeased with the limited and unpleasant options available to my patients in the past, and I fervently hoped that better, far-reaching alternatives would someday be attainable. Now, thankfully, they are. But you have to take control of the situation by admitting to the problem, examining its probable causes, and seeking treatment.

The earlier the intervention, the better the result will be. If ED is something you worry about or have already experienced, whether it is occasional or more frequent, help is now available. Remember: ED has a profound effect on the lives of the people it touches. Countless marriages and long-term relationships have been broken by it; people who otherwise deeply cared for each other felt separation was a better solution; and innumerable others continued to live together sexually unfulfilled. Sex is, of course, not the only component of a strong and lasting relationship, but I believe it is an important one. And if ED is a problem, the new drugs will not only treat it, they will help you renew your bond to the person you care about.

The Search for a Miracle Cure

UNTIL NOW, THE treatment of ED and the ceaseless quest for its cure has been an intriguing story of conjecture, myth, and a lot of trial—and error. Ironically, the medical research of this century, most of which has been male-oriented, has failed to focus on one of the few maladies unique to males. Even worse, the problem has been treated crudely and bluntly, without an effort to find an easy-to-take medication, and with complete disregard for the quality of a man's life. I repeat: until now.

It's extraordinary. The hearts of tens of thousands of men have been studied so that the proper pills, along with behavioral changes, could make them, or keep them, healthy. Their cholesterol counts have been measured millions of times, so that the correct dosage of drugs to counter potentially life-threatening conditions could be administered. Blood pressures have been taken endlessly in order to save lives with medications. Still, when it came to the issue of a consistently firm erection—a fundamental core of masculine identity—the reaction was one of indifference. Millions of men were told the problem was in their heads and that mainstream medicine had no answer. In fact, when I attended medical school only twenty-five years ago, erectile dysfunction was not a subject that was examined or discussed at length.

Why?

Because sexuality—and erectile problems in particular—were never fully regarded as an appropriate or urgent medical subject, much less an essential part of health and well-being. As a result, research that focused on male sexual functioning lagged far behind inquiries into other areas of medicine.

In my own practice, sexual medicine was one area that was difficult to integrate into the medical overview of my male patients. This was particularly frustrating, since internal medicine focuses on the health of the whole patient, not just on a singular organ or disease. I could help the women who came to see me about their sexual problems by referring them to experts who handled their particular concerns. But not for men. The reasons were twofold: first, the majority of men didn't speak about their ED, and second, the available solutions were few and far from satisfactory.

There were times when even I thought that ED was a condition that the patient could control himself. The prevailing "wisdom" of the time, I'm embarrassed to say, was that it required some kind of behavior modification, similar to obesity treatment. I hoped that someday a miracle cure would come along to help these men. Not only would it alleviate their anxiety and frustration, it would lift a lot of responsibility off the medical establishment, which didn't know how to help them.

That miracle cure was something that eluded us for a very long time.

A Look Back for a Cure

ED has always been with us; treatments have been employed to combat it for thousands of years. Not surprisingly, the view of the problem, as well as the remedies for it, grows out of the culture and belief system of a particular time.

To fully understand how far back erectile problems go, we need only look to the Bible. In Genesis, ED is regarded as a punishment for committing adultery. Abimelech was stricken with it after just *thinking* about having sex with Abraham's wife. Two thousand years ago, the Egyptians, a sophisticated and innovative people, recorded their recipes to cure ED. In their culture, it was attributed to the wrath of a particular god, and a typical corrective included pacifying the appropriate idol with offerings. At other times, herbal enhancers were used to restore diminished or lost virility.

The ancient Greeks were also no strangers to ED. At that time, it was commonly believed that a vast array of erectile problems would be experienced by any man who, as a child, had sat on a tomb. The cure was to drink a potion made with the scrapings of a knife used to geld rams.

Interestingly, the very first references to the psychological roots of ED can be traced all the way back to the Greek legend of Iphiclus. As a youth, Iphiclus, the son of King Phylacus, saw his father coming toward him clutching the handle of a bloody knife that had been used to castrate a ram. Terrified by the thought that his father would turn on him with the weapon, Iphiclus soon developed chronic erectile failure. A physician named Melampus figured out a way to help him with a technique later commonly employed in psychiatry. He showed the prince the gelding knife. When he observed that the blood was long dried and the knife itself rusted, Iphiclus was able to overcome his fear and his ED disappeared.

As time went on, most men weren't as fortunate as the young Greek. By the Middle Ages, the Catholic Church attributed ED to witchcraft, as well as to the effects of demonic possession. A sexual hex known as a "ligature" was commonly used to invoke ED in an unsuspecting foe through the power of suggestion. All the instigator had to do was tie a series of knots in a cord or a strip of leather and hide it in a secret place. He would then let his victim know what he'd done. Depending on both the number and specific configuration of knots, it was believed the victim would then develop partial or total erectile failure. In some cases, total sterility could, it was thought, be achieved. Of course, hexes relied heavily on the belief in magic. If a man accepted their power, he could be influenced by them. Conversely, if he felt that an incantation could actually break the spell, he might achieve some positive results.

Folk medicine has always been applied whenever a man's virility showed signs of waning. A seemingly endless succession of herbal potions, drugs, and mechanical devices has been employed over the centuries, from crushed rhinoceros horn and pulverized antelope, deer, and horse testicles, to parings of human nails. In times of desperation, a piece of bone was actually eased into the urethra to stiffen the penis.

The mandrake plant, a member of the nightshade family, was used extensively in medieval Europe, northern Africa, and Asia as both a painkiller and a cure for ED. It is even mentioned in the Old Testament, under the name "dudaim," as the stimulant used by Jacob. Stemless, with bell-shaped flowers, the plant's long and thick root, which often divides into two sections, resembles the lower male torso. It contains many alkaloids of medicinal value, making it one of the most discussed plants in medical literature, as well as the subject of myth and superstition. Alkaloids are a diverse group of nitrogen-containing substances produced by plants that have powerful effects on body function; some of the more common alkaloids include atropine, morphine, quinine, and codeine.

And then there was food. Throughout history, edibles, especially those phallic in shape, were employed as virility boosters. Asparagus, bananas, carrots, and cucumbers stood out in this category. Some indigenous tribes in coastal areas traditionally rubbed long, slender fish against their penises in the hope that they would become similarly long and hard.

The Beginning of Medical Science

By the sixteenth century, a degree of science had been introduced into the study of male sexual function. Varolio, an Italian physician, was the first to note that blood flowed through the penis. Unfortunately, this keen insight was followed by a gap in medical research that can be attributed to prudish societal attitudes about anything remotely sexual. In fact, it wasn't until two hundred years later that physicians made the next significant observation about ED: it had at least one physical cause. Even more importantly, they figured out how to treat it successfully.

This stunning event was centered around King Louis XVI of France. In 1770, when he was sixteen, Louis was unable to achieve intercourse with his wife, Marie Antoinette. It is said that he suffered from total erectile dysfunction. Where royalty was concerned, ED was an especially thorny problem. Dynasties needed heirs. So Louis consulted with the medical experts of his day and a diagnosis was made. It seemed that the main cause of his problem was an excessively tight foreskin. Following a successful circumcision—several years after his arranged marriage—he was finally able to perform sexually. Eventually, he fathered two children.

In this country, however, treatments for ED—such as they were—still tended to be based on folk medicine. One old American recipe for a sexual salve combined thorn apple, black pepper, and honey. This mix was applied to the penis before intercourse. The thorn apple is now known to contain atropine and hyoscine, two strong alkaloids. Absorbed through the mucous membrane of the penis, they may have helped to trigger an erection. The pepper, which produces a burning sensation, would have helped to maintain it. The honey, however, acted solely as a lubricant.

Another natural remedy for ED used since the 1870s included the leaves of the damiana plant (*Turnera diffusa*), a small shrub found in desert areas. An herbal tincture made from the plant's tannin and volatile oils became popular in the southwest United States and Mexico as a sexual enhancer. It's believed that the damiana irritates the urethra slightly, thereby expanding the sensitivity of the penis.

Jimsonweed (*Datura stramonium*), originally named Jamestown weed, was regularly used by Native Americans as an erection builder. A tall, highly poisonous plant that is also a member of the nightshade family, its seeds were powdered, mixed with butter, and eaten; for added measure, the mixture was smeared on the genitals. The recipe was certainly time-honored: jimsonweed is mentioned in Homer's *Odyssey* as well as two works by Shakespeare: *Romeo and Juliet* and *Antony and Cleopatra*. Over the years, this flowering plant has acquired many other names, including locoweed, devil's apple, devil's weed, angel tulip, and stinkweed. It's readily absorbed through all mucous membranes and excreted mainly by the kidneys. All parts of the jimsonweed are toxic; as little as one-half teaspoon of the seeds has been reported to cause death from cardiac and pulmonary arrest.

In this century, a major theme emerged from what little ongoing ED research was taking place. Sigmund Freud, along with his fellow psychiatrists, emphasized the contribution of psychogenic factors, often childhood experiences, that led to ED. With a psychiatrist's help, the patient would recall these traumatic episodes in the belief that their acknowledgment would resolve any erectile problems. Unfortunately, this process, long and arduous, could go on for years, while the man in question still suffered from ED. This powerful concept, which influenced both the definition of the problem and its treatment, was regarded as gospel until as recently as the 1980s.

OTHER CULTURES, OTHER CURES

The Chinese began using ginseng as a sex booster five thousand years ago. Ginseng, which means "man root," most likely earned its early reputation for enhancing male sexuality from its distinctly human-looking shape. Ancient Chinese writings tell us that ginseng has long been used to prevent and cure a broad range of ailments, including ED. In India, ancient Vedic texts relate that the root will impart the power of a bull to men young and old. In fact, ginseng does seem to have a sexual-stimulating ability. Today, a substantial body of medical literature, published primarily in China, Japan, Korea, and Russia, supports traditional beliefs about the sexual effectiveness of this root.

There are three major varieties of ginseng: American, Panax, and Siberian, each with a specific use. It's the Panax variety, also known as Asian ginseng, that has played a major role in producing erections naturally without complications. This type of ginseng comes in two forms: white and red. The colors relate to the particular method employed to preserve the root. Red ginseng, considered the more powerful of the two, is usually given to people who are lacking energy. In 1995, a study of ninety patients was carried out at the Yonsei University College of Medicine in Seoul, South Korea, and a report on the study in the *International Journal of Impotency Research* stated that those men taking red ginseng had significantly strengthened penile rigidity and girth, as well as heightened libido and increased pleasure. Their degree of satisfaction outweighed that of patients who received either a placebo or a low dose of trazodone, an antidepressant with positive prosexual capabilities. Investigation of this fascinating root is ongoing.

Research on cantharides, or Spanish fly, on the other hand, has completely stopped—with good reason. Wildly touted over centuries as both an erection intensifier and a love potion, this powder is made by crushing the dried meloid beetle, an insect readily found in parts of the Mediterranean. While the powder may produce a warm, sometimes burning sensation in the penis after ingestion, it is, in fact, totally useless in inducing an erection. Too much of the substance can actually damage the urinary and digestive tracts—and a mere one thousandth of an ounce is enough to destroy the kidneys. Given its extreme toxicity, true Spanish fly is now listed as a Class 1 poison and is unavailable in the United States.

An herb obtained from the inner bark of the yohimbe, an evergreen tree that grows in Cameroon, Congo, and Gabon, has also been used by Africans to boost sexual prowess. Yohimbine, the active ingredient of yohimbe bark, is a natural ingredient that causes an increase in small blood vessel dilation. The enlargement of vessels increases blood flow to the penis, leading to an erection. Men given yohimbine intravenously have been known to have almost instant erections. Interestingly, however, when yohimbine is injected directly into the penis there is no resulting erection. This finding has led some researchers to speculate that yohimbine is actually affecting the pleasure centers in the brain—and a specific neurotransmitter, dopamine, in particular. The herb may also be influencing the blood levels of norepinephrine, a neurotransmitter or brain chemical that stimulates the sex center located in the hypothalamus.

Yohimbine is still used by many urologists to treat ED. While it can take up to three weeks before results are noticeable, the herb is particularly effective for men without any sexual difficulties, but who seek enhanced pleasure. Not only does it have the ability to augment libido, it can stimulate erections and trigger more powerful orgasms.

And There Was Always Alcohol

For centuries, people have believed that alcohol eases the way toward an erection because of its powerful effect on mood. And while it is true that moderate consumption—a glass of wine, a bottle of beer—can help to lessen sexual inhibition and intensify libido, excessive amounts produce the opposite effect. The reason is linked to the way alcohol acts in the human body, especially in the central nervous system. The drinker will first feel a dual sensation of ease and exhilaration, but it is brief. As blood alcohol content rises, there is progressive impairment to judgment, memory, and sensory perception. And when it comes to sex, the truth is that alcohol's impact on the central nervous system often results in a canceled performance.

When moderate social drinking turns to excessive drinking, or alcoholism, the nerves that control erectile function become impaired. Combining heavy drinking with smoking, the use of illicit drugs, over-eating, stress, or high blood pressure intensifies ED problems even further.

My Journey into Sexual Medicine

The desperate need for a quick, effective solution for ED was brought home to me by the action of one of my patients. It's a case that I cannot forget. Miles, a quiet man with a gentle manner, was in his late thirties when he first came to see me more than fifteen years ago. I met him when I treated his wife, Kathleen, for pneumonia. The father of three and very successful in his work, he was in fine health. His only complaint—if it could actually be called that—was of general fatigue. His zest for life, he told me, had waned.

Concerned that these were warning signs of a general depression,

I asked if his feelings were linked to any singular event or change in circumstance. His answer was an unemotional no; he said that he probably had been working too hard, and that it was getting to him. But over the course of his twice-a-year visits, his malaise never lifted. Eventually, I suggested that he consult a psychiatrist. But he didn't feel it was necessary.

However, he did tell me something new. From time to time he had trouble getting an erection. I recited to him what I had been taught: his problem was in the realm of psychiatry, not internal medicine. I actually quoted the set-in-stone statistics that all doctors at the time knew by heart: "Almost 90 percent of sexual problems are psychological in nature." With that, I offered the names of several highly regarded experts, and Miles said he would consider seeking out one of them. That was the first—and last—time that he ever mentioned his problem.

A few months after his visit, I received a frantic call from Kathleen, who asked me to meet her at the emergency room of a local hospital. Miles had taken an overdose of pills. When I arrived, the news was terrible. He had already died.

Eventually, Kathleen told me the series of events that led to this tragedy. The sad truth was that Miles took his own life, in part, because of a growing despondency over his inability to function sexually. Kathleen felt that losing his erections had led to diminished self-esteem and, ultimately, to a total loss of self. His sense of failure was so acute that he felt he could no longer be a father to his children, or a husband to his wife. His personal worth had been so devalued that, for him, there was no other recourse.

Miles's case haunted me for a long time. I wondered what pieces of the puzzle I had missed and how I could have intervened. He had told me that there was a lot of work-related stress in his life. Was that the cause of his ED, I wondered?

I realized that Miles was probably only one of millions of men who suffered alone. There had to be a way to bring help to those who needed it. But before that could happen, I had to find out everything I could about penile physiology, the workings of male sexual organs, and what the available treatments entailed. I consulted colleagues whose specialties were in urology, psychiatry, psychology, and sex therapy. I met with physicians who were treating patients suffering from prostate cancer and diabetes.

The first—and the most startling—thing I learned was that in addition to psychiatric treatment, there were only three basic medical procedures to alleviate ED: vacuum erection therapy, penile injection therapy, and penile implant surgery.

The Methods of the Twentieth Century

Vacuum erection therapy was developed in 1961 by Geddings Osbon. A sufferer of ED, he refused to accept the fact that he could no longer have sexual intimacy with his wife of three decades. Working intently for the next couple of years, he invented a plastic device, actually an external vacuum, that was capable of inducing an erection. A reversible, noninvasive form of dealing with ED, the vacuum device was used by Osbon for more than twenty years. In 1983, he was awarded a patent for it. The company he founded, Osbon Medical Systems, still manufactures and distributes his Erecaid vacuum device worldwide.

The device acts in a very simple way. When a man wants to have an erection, he places a clear plastic cylinder over his penis, and either a manual or special electrical pump is used to create negative pressure in the tube. Regardless of the source of the erection problem, this pressure causes vessels in the penis to fill with blood, just as they would in a normal erection. Once an erection is achieved—it may take two minutes or so—a flexible tension ring is slipped off the bottom of the cylinder around the base of the penis to keep blood from flowing out of the penis, thereby allowing it to stay hard when the cylinder is removed. The resulting erection may be safely sustained for at least thirty minutes. Allowing the erection to last longer than that can produce damage to delicate erectile tissue.

The pump does have several advantages, the primary ones being that it is very safe and free of side effects. And it can be utilized whenever an erection is desired. Some urologists are now recommending pump use following prostate and penile surgery to promote erections and thereby protect the penis from potential damage caused by the lack of regularly occurring nocturnal erections.

In day-to-day use, some pump users complain that their penis feels numb, or that it becomes discolored, misshapen, and cold to the touch. Many speak of the interruption of intimacy that using it brings during lovemaking. Research shows that about 7 percent of men using it experience mild discomfort upon ejaculation or varying degrees of ejaculation impairment. The pump costs between $400 to $500 and is available only with a physician's prescription.

Penile injection therapy came about by chance. In 1980, the French physician Ronald Virag reported that during surgery on the penis, he inadvertently injected an anesthetized patient in the wrong part of the penis with papaverine, a nitrogen-containing substance derived from the opium poppy. The resulting relaxation of the smooth muscle of the penile arterial walls created an unexpected two-hour erection. The mistake by Virag set in motion serious research into the use of injectable medication for relief of ED.

At around the same time, Giles Brindley, a British physiologist and research scientist, found that when the drug phenoxybenzamine was injected directly into the corpora cavernosa of the penis, an erection could be produced within a few minutes. Still, even though it was a powerful substance, phenoxybenzamine had serious side effects, including cardiac arrhythmia, nausea, and hyperventilation. Additionally, it was found to be carcinogenic in test animals.

In 1984, in Paris, a New York urologist, Dr. Adrian Zorgniotti, presented his first case studies of self-injection using a dual combination of papaverine and phentolamine. The latter drug interrupts the passage of neurotransmitters, which then causes relaxation of the smooth muscles of the penis. Two years later, Japanese researchers presented evidence that injections of prostaglandin E-1 produced powerful erections. Finally, modern medicine had injectable drugs that, used either alone or in combination, were able to give a man an erection whenever he wanted one. Slowly, news of the favorable results with the injectable medication began to spread within the small international community of urologists who were treating ED. Most began utilizing all three—papaverine, phentolamine, and prostaglandin E-1—in what was referred to as "tri-mix."

HOW THE DRUGS WORK

The specific formulation of tri-mix drugs to be administered is based on the type of erection achieved with test dosages. This is determined by your urologist during an office visit in which a sample tri-mix formulation is injected into the penis. Your comfort, the degree of erection obtained, and the time it takes for you to lose the erection are carefully observed by the doctor. The usual dose of phentolamine can range from 0.5 to 1 milligram (mg); 30 mg or less for papaverine; and 5 to 40 micrograms (mcg) for prostaglandin E-1.

After the exact dosage is determined, the doctor has the medication compounded (prepared) at a special pharmacy. He also has to teach his patient how to self-inject. Understandably, this might take some getting used to, since the medication is shot into the base of the penis with a small hypodermic syringe. While this certainly sounds painful, some men describe it as merely a mild pinching sensation.

After receiving the dose, the man will achieve an erection within five to twenty minutes, the result of the relaxation of smooth muscle tissue, the dilation of main arteries, and blood filling the penis. The erection can last between thirty and ninety minutes, becoming more rigid with sexual stimulation. However, the erection does not always disappear immediately after orgasm or ejaculation. While the injections have a high success rate—over 70 percent—the main cause of failure is usually due to the drugs' inability to override poor blood flow to the penis. In some cases, although the tri-mix produces an initial erection, damaged veins in the penis allow blood to escape rapidly, resulting in an unsustainable erection.

To be certain that the appropriate dosage has been created for you, your erection should be over by the time you leave the doctor's office. If too much is administered, priapism, an unwanted, prolonged erection that lasts for three or four hours, can develop. This painful and dangerous medical condition—named for Priapus, the Greek god of procreation—can lead to the destruction of erectile tissue if left untreated. Thankfully, it can be reversed by injecting an adrenaline-like drug into the penis.

Not surprisingly, the actual pain caused from injecting the drugs into the penis, as well as the mere thought of doing so, is enough to turn many men away from the procedure. In reality, the injection itself is not painful but rather it's the injected prostaglandin medication—reacting with nerve-damaged and blood-deprived tissue—that actually triggers the pain.

Although approximately 500,000 men seek this treatment each year—which costs about $7 per shot—half reject it before the year is over. One 1990 study found that 51 percent of the group dropped out after receiving just one test shot. The average patient, however, stayed in the group for seven months before leaving it. However, urologists find that those who continue with long-term use of the injectables had overcome resistance to self-injection early on and made a smooth transition to injection therapy. Some experts believe that success rate may be linked to detailed instruction from the doctor or trained medical personnel in mastering the injection technique so that the patient feels competent and comfortable in self-administration of the drugs.

Now, there is another injectable option which uses yet a different medication. This 1996 FDA-approved prescription drug is called Caverject and is more expensive than tri-mix, at $20 to $25 for each injection. The drug comes in two strengths in a disposable, single-dose syringe that's prefilled with the medication alprostadil, an effective erection-enhancing agent. Injected directly into the base of the penis five minutes before a sexual encounter, the drug increases blood flow, producing an eventual erection. Although Medicare does not pay for injection therapy, some insurance plans do.

Still another "injectable" became available in 1997. MUSE, developed by a new California company called Vivus, employs a small, specially designed plastic plunger that is placed at the tip of the penis. Once the plunger is pressed in, a tiny, rice-size pellet of alprostadil is pushed into the urethra. There, moisture left by urine causes the pellet to dissolve, triggering an erection minutes later.

Certainly less invasive than a hypodermic injection of medication, MUSE is still far from being the perfect virility solution because it creates an artificial erection in the absence of a partner's sexual stimulus. Also, many men complain of a burning pain in the penis after insertion of the drug. As with the injectable tri-mix, your doctor needs to titrate the correct dosage of MUSE for you. Some men may require double or triple the standard dose, while others are so sensitive to the medication that they have fainted with the lowest test dose. I advise you not to change dosages on your own at home.

Some men are dissatisfied with the overall effect of the pellet on erections. One patient actually described his penis as resembling "a snake that swallowed a mouse. My penis was large and hard at the top, where the medication had dissolved, but farther back it was soft and wobbly. When my wife and I wanted to have sex I had to stuff my dick in, instead of thrusting it. It was frustrating—in every way."

Still, even with the not-so-perfect nature of the drug, some urologists feel there is a place for MUSE in an ED treatment program. "I find that if a man has not used any of the other therapies," said New York urologist Dr. Eli Lizza, "then if he tries MUSE, he is often satisfied with the results." Judging by the early response to the medication, many men were certainly interested in trying the drug. The entire first year's supply of the drug sold out within three weeks after being introduced to the market and the company had difficulty keeping up with the unexpected demand.

Penile implant surgery was generally used in older patients who had the procedure performed prior to the availability of injectable medications. The prosthetic device is costly—between $12,000 and $15,000. For men whose sex lives had been drastically impaired due to diabetes, radical pelvic surgery to treat prostate cancer, severe bladder or colon problems, or physical injury to the penis, the implant was often the only option.

There are two basic types of penile implants: inflatable, of which several types are available, and malleable semirigid. The surgery involves placing a pair of rods or cylinders in the penis. Extremely compact, the hollow cylinders, which come in a variety of widths and lengths, are implanted next to the corpora cavernosa. A small container that holds fluid for the cylinders is situated in the lower part of the abdomen and a pump is inserted in the scrotum. Whenever an erection is desired, the man squeezes the pump several times, which transfers the fluid from the container to the inflatable cylinders, which then expand, widening and lengthening the penis. To stop the erection, the valve at the top of the pump is squeezed and the fluid returns to the abdominal reservoir, causing penile flaccidity.

The inflatable implant has the significant advantage of allowing a man to instantly get an erection. The disadvantage is its complexity. The apparatus is so mechanically complex that when a problem occurs surgery is needed to fix it. Other drawbacks include post-surgical discomfort; many men experience severe penile and abdominal pain for up to six weeks following implantation.

The malleable semirigid implant consists of two silicone rods that can easily be bent or straightened. Once surgically implanted in the corpora cavernosa, a man will have a permanent erection. Bending the rods so that the penis is close to the body hides it, while straightening the organ with one or two fingers immediately readies it for intercourse.

While the device is simple to use, it does have its limitations. In the case of either implantation, infection can occur. In that event, the implants have to be removed. Depending on the degree of penile tissue damage, another implant may be reinserted after sufficient healing. However, scarring may be so severe that it can rule out a subsequent reimplant—permanently leaving the man without any possibility of intercourse.

ONE PATIENT'S STORY

Just three options to treat ED—all with side effects or considerable disadvantages—were certainly better than none. But they were hardly optimal and imposed numerous restrictions on men.

That was the case with Frank. Back in 1989, I began to treat this forty-five-year-old's atherosclerosis, the sticky plaque that forms in the arteries, eventually clogging them and obstructing blood flow. With a cholesterol count of 260, there was cause for concern; Frank had to be monitored to prevent heart disease. However, there was another matter as well. One of the primary indicators of atherosclerosis is a diminishing of erectile function, and I asked Frank if this was the case with him.

Initially taken aback, he blurted out, "How did you know?" And while it was, at first, difficult for him to speak about his problem, he eventually grew more comfortable as we talked.

"There *are* options for you," I told him. But we were both aware that for Frank, who wasn't in a relationship, the situation was a difficult and frustrating one. For one thing, his increasing inability to have an erection was extremely disturbing. For another, the treatment choices were so off-putting that he was concerned that they would turn away any potential partner.

The first thing Frank tried was the vacuum pump. While it reliably produced an erection and was effective, after several months he gave it up. He felt that there just wasn't a way to successfully introduce it into a romantic setting. For him it was humiliating, and just drew attention to his physical limitations.

Then I suggested that he use tri-mix. Much less "mechanical" than the pump, he could administer the shot in the bathroom, out of sight. He tried it several times but was disappointed once again.

"Let me ask you a question," Frank challenged me after he gave up tri-mix. "How would you like to treat an ongoing headache, one that puts a stop to your life and makes you feel miserable, with an injection in your head? What if every time your head hurt you'd have to excuse yourself and go into the bathroom to plunge medication behind your eye? How would *you* feel about it?"

I confessed that I wouldn't like it at all.

"And forget about spontaneity and romance," he continued. "I feel like a machine waiting for a fuel-up. I used to think that stopping to put on a condom was intrusive—little did I know. These treatments may work physically, but they sure as hell don't work emotionally—either for me or for the women I'm interested in. You give me pills for my cholesterol, why can't you do the same for my ED?"

Frank's frustration hit me. The problem was not only in the limited options for treatment, but in their detachment from the man using them. They were, at best, solutions born of physical necessity. But no one, it seemed, was taking into consideration the emotional aspects of treatment, much less an easy-to-use, successful remedy.

THE BIRTH OF SEXUAL MEDICINE

The first steps leading to a better remedy for ED—an oral one—were taken by Dr. Adrian Zorgniotti. By 1990, I was referring all of my ED patients to this pioneering physician who had dedicated the bulk of his medical career to unraveling the mysteries of erectile dysfunction. Dr. Zorgniotti believed that ED had an overwhelming physical cause. With penile implants as the only viable treatment, even for men with minimal ED, his goal had been to find a way to get the short-circuited penis fully functional, quickly and easily. It was Dr. Zorgniotti who was one of the first doctors to combine the use of two drugs, phentolamine and papaverine, into an intercavernous injection that would help open up the blood vessels of the penis.

"Adrian was a true pioneer in the field of ED," recalled Dr. Eli Lizza, who in 1988 as a young urological microsurgeon had been invited to work closely with Dr. Zorgniotti. "He was a visionary who was never satisfied with the options at his disposal. He always tried to go a step beyond and find out how he could expand the field.

"His injection therapy became extremely popular and he had patients from around the world," said Dr. Lizza. "But to a man, each one asked if a pill would ever be available to bring on an erection."

Dr. Zorgniotti was aware of the specific side effect of a drug which had been commonly used in the United States for over forty years to regulate high blood pressure. Regitine, or phentolamine mesylate, was known to stimulate erections in many of the men who took it. However, no one had been able to develop an oral medication with phentolamine that could aid men with ED.

"Adrian saw a need to fill and decided he was the man to fill it," said Dr. Lizza, who now shared an office in a town house on 74th Street in Manhattan with Dr. Zorgniotti. Working in the basement laboratory of the town house with medication purchased from a pharmaceutical company, Dr. Zorgniotti would make his own phentolamine pills, mixing the powdered drug with a starch filler and pressing them out one by one into either 25 mg- or 50 mg-strength pills.

In 1993, Dr. Zorgniotti administered 50 mg of his phentolamine tablets to eighty-five men whose ED had various causes. The results were extremely promising. Comparing them to a group of men taking 5 mg of phenoxybenzamine capsules, Dr. Zorgniotti found that 42 percent of the patients using the phentolamine were able to achieve erections sufficient for vaginal penetration. The major drawback, however, was that the drug took at least ninety minutes to work, thereby putting a severe crimp on the possibility of spontaneity in lovemaking.

Undeterred, Dr. Zorgniotti developed a new delivery system the following year using a buccal, or oral, solution of 20 mg of phentolamine mesylate. This medication in pill form was held in the mouth until fully dissolved. In yet another study, he formulated a filter strip soaked with the liquid drug, which was then placed between the cheek and gum, where the medication was absorbed quickly into the bloodstream. Tested on sixty-nine men, along with a placebo group, the outcome was significant: more than 32 percent of the men responded to the phentolamine mesylate with a full erection. Even more impressive was the fact that the reaction took place within twenty minutes. While this drug was costly and not easily obtainable, it was yet another of Dr. Zorgniotti's breakthroughs in the development of a new kind of treatment for ED.

Sadly, Dr. Zorgniotti died in 1994 from the complications of severe adult onset diabetes before he was able to finish the final phase of his work. He was sixty-eight years old. "He was a mentor to me," said Dr. Lizza. "I lost his friendship and counsel. The medical world lost a giant."

FOLLOWING IN THE FOOTSTEPS

Fortunately, however, with Dr. Zorgniotti's newest breakthrough, it was now possible for me and other doctors to prescribe a compounded version of his pills. Working with a compounding pharmacist (a druggist who prepares medications himself, as opposed to one who dispenses ready-made drugs), I was able to offer the phentolamine pills in buccal form that were custom-tailored to the varied needs of my patients. I started them with the lowest dose, 20 mg. If that didn't achieve the optimal result, I increased the dosage incrementally until a satisfactory erection was achieved. Unfortunately, such a regimen of drug therapy was costly. Each pill cost approximately $35.

Finally, there was a method to treat ED effectively—from both a physical and psychological point of view. It had become apparent from the favorable outcome in patients using the buccal pills that restoring erectile function was just one aspect of the treatment of ED. With this more natural approach, the pills seemed to facilitate a release from the stress and anxiety that ED brings on. I realized that a cure for ED would have a profound effect beyond the immediate physical one. The buccal pills had already indicated that by:

- ensuring spontaneity in lovemaking
- aiding in the reentry to a functioning sexual life
- permitting patients an opportunity to mend relationships that may have been damaged by ED
- enabling partners to work together in the most natural way possible to restore trust and sexual gratification

In addition, having become familiar with many of the underlying physical causes of erection problems, I realized that the entire health of a man had to be taken into consideration when treating ED. That's when the components of my virility-enhancement program—which include specific diet and supplement recommendations, along with an exercise regimen and instructions on relieving stress—began to fall into place. But to fully appreciate why I built an entire program around the treatment of ED, it's crucial to understand the mechanics of erection, as well as the components which contribute to good penile health.

THE MECHANICS OF ERECTION

An erection is dependent upon the finely orchestrated actions of muscles, nerves, and blood vessels in the penis. Additionally, it requires good blood flow, which is regulated by the nervous system, to bring about the hydraulic, or lifting, action.

Three to six spontaneous erections occur without erotic stimulation every night during REM (rapid eye movement), or dream, sleep. Erections which take place during normal sexual activity, however, begin in the male's conscious brain with a nervous system response to either real or imagined erotic stimulation. The change in the penis from flaccid (soft) to tumescent (swollen) to erect (rigid) is caused by an intricate partnership involving the brain, blood vessels, nerves, and hormones.

The shaft of the penis holds two individual chambers called the corpora cavernosa. A spongy tissue constructed of thousands of expandable saclike structures fills the chambers, which extend from the base to the tip of the organ. This tissue also contains blood vessels and smooth muscles. The urethra, the channel for urine and ejaculate, runs on the underside of the corpora cavernosa, while a membrane, known as the tunica albuginea, surrounds the corpora. In the normal, flaccid state, the smooth muscle keeps the blood vessels constricted, keeping blood out and the penis soft.

An erection begins when the brain senses something arousing.

Impulses are then sent from the brain to the lower part of the back, through the pelvis, and to the penis. Nerve stimulation, most likely induced by nitric oxide, a gaseous molecule, causes the smooth muscles of the penis to relax. This allows increased quantities of blood to flow in through the right and left cavernosal arteries, filling the space within the cavernosa. For the blood to fill the penis and cause it to become longer, wider, and harder, it has to multiply to about six times its normal flow. Like a sponge, the corpora tissues quickly expand with blood, engorging and enlarging the penis.

Then, as the corpora cavernosa continue to swell, they press against the veins that normally allow blood to flow out, effectively preventing it from leaving. The tunica albuginea also helps to trap blood there, with the result that pressure is built. Finally, packed with blood, the corpora become rigid and erect, making the penis firm enough for penetration. As long as the inflow of blood is maintained, and the outflow is prevented, the erection will be sustained.

All of these actions happen automatically; men have no voluntary control over these mechanical forces.

When the Mechanism Breaks Down

There are many things that can interfere and prevent an erection from happening, or can keep an erect penis from maintaining its rigidity. The physical problems that are known to cause ED include:

- vascular problems, resulting in blocked arteries
- nerve disorders
- vein trouble
- medications
- other causes

Vascular Problems

The major cause of erectile difficulties I have seen typically originate from problems with the two tiny, deep cavernosal arteries. These blood vessels are about as wide as the tip of a pencil. A man who is experiencing vascular problems will typically find that his erection has become less firm. He'll start out with a strong erection, but during sexual activity it will suddenly begin to lose rigidity. Over time, he'll begin to experience difficulty in having an erection at all.

What has happened in many cases is diffuse blockage to both arteries, caused by fatty deposits. This process begins when men are in their twenties, and is mostly due to high-fat diets, hereditary conditions, high cholesterol, or, sometimes, a combination of the three factors. As the blockage slowly progresses, the arteries are unable to dilate enough to permit increased blood flow to the penis.

Often, the types of blockages which contribute to the early stages of ED are the first early warning signs of mounting vascular problems that lead to cardiovascular disease. Problems in the small erectile arteries can indicate that there are serious blockages in larger blood vessels, too, especially those to the heart or brain. One recent study found that there was a 25 percent incidence of heart attack or stroke in the two years following the onset of ED.

Nerve Disorders

ED can be experienced when there are problems with the nerves that are responsible for erections. The nerves are signal carriers, relaying information from the brain to the penile arteries. Alerted, the blood vessels open, allowing enough blood to rush in to cause hardness. If, however, there is a problem with these nerves, either from spinal cord, brain, prostate, or groin injuries, the messages aren't transmitted correctly. The outcome is an impaired erection—or none at all.

The major nerve problem is produced by diabetes mellitus, a chronic disorder usually caused by a deficient secretion of insulin, the hormonal substance manufactured by the endocrine glands in the pancreas. It is now estimated that the prevalence of ED in men with diabetes is between 35 percent and 75 percent. More than half of them notice the first onset of ED within ten years of developing the disease.

Genetic predisposition, along with obesity, are the most significant factors known to trigger diabetes. In either case, the condition adversely affects the nerves, making it progressively more difficult for nerve impulses to reach the penis. In some cases, diabetes delivers a double threat: it can also damage blood vessels, causing them to become blocked and interrupt blood flow to the penis.

Multiple sclerosis, a progressive nervous system disorder, and Parkinson's disease, a degenerative brain syndrome, also create neurological disturbances that can lead to ED. Other nerve disruptions can be brought on by back surgery, as well as disk herniation in the lower back. (If a patient tells me his erections were normal before sustaining a back injury, I immediately suspect nerve damage.) Other sources include cancer surgery or any radiation therapy on the pelvic area. If the prostate gland is removed, or an operation is performed to remove cancer in the lower rectum or colon, delicate nerves can also be damaged, leading to erection problems.

Vein Trouble

For an erection to occur, the veins that carry the blood from the penis must shut down, trapping the blood in the two chambers. If the veins don't close, the blood, obviously, will run out. The analogy is like running water in a sink with an open drain. No matter how much water flows in, nothing is stopping it from continuing on. Thankfully, this is a very rare problem. Even an ED specialist, who may see hundreds of cases a year, will, typically, only see fewer than ten men with vein trouble. To date, surgery on the veins and arteries of the penis has not been very successful.

Medications

Many times, ED is a side effect of taking a drug. The most common offenders are prescription drugs for high blood pressure, heart ailments, and allergies. Medications used to combat depression, especially the selective serotonin-reuptake inhibitors (SSRIs), such as Prozac, Zoloft, and Paxil, can also be the culprits.

Frequently, if a man is taking more than one medication, the damaging effects are cumulative. For example, I have seen cases where a patient is taking a drug for his depression, and, while he is experiencing some difficulty maintaining an erection, he can still have sex. However, if a second medication, say for hypertension, is added, his sexual performance will be severely impaired. A complete loss of erectile function can result.

The men in these predicaments have sex lives held hostage by the very medications that can save them. It's an ironic and frustrating situation to be in. I have seen men blame themselves, or their partners, when they weren't even aware that their problems had a physiological cause.

Sometimes, men will suspect that the medication mix is responsible for, or contributing to, their ED. On their own, they may decide to try lowered dosages or stop taking the drugs altogether. This very dangerous action can be deadly and must be avoided. In the case of hypertensive medication, lack of the drug may cause blood pressure to suddenly soar to dangerously high levels. The outcome can be a stroke or a heart attack.

Right now, there are more than two hundred medications on the market that can seriously compromise erections and sexual performance. Unfortunately, the Food and Drug Administration, the government agency that approves all medications, doesn't require pharmaceutical companies to reduce potential sexual side effects. But then, men rarely voice their concerns about something as personal as diminished sexual performance. Therefore, reporting erection difficulties brought about by a particular medication to a physician is a rare event. Many doctors aren't even aware of the problem their prescriptions are causing. And, for those men who do seek help from their doctors, the frequent recommendation is for them to get psychological counseling, which leaves them, as far as treatment for their ED is concerned, back in the middle of the twentieth century.

When it comes to avoiding certain medications because of their effect on sexual response, there is no simple answer. Not every drug will give each man who uses it trouble. If you suddenly notice that you are having erection problems where none existed before, take a good look at any and all medications that you are using.

Other Causes

Removal of the prostate can affect the ability to have an erection. This is the invariable result of the most commonly performed procedure, known as the radical prostatectomy. A newer surgical technique now attempts to preserve the appropriate nerves in order to safeguard erectile function. However, 50 percent of the men will experience erectile difficulties, even with this technique. Hopefully, improvements in this technique and newer surgical procedures will be able to reduce the incidence of postsurgical erectile problems.

Testosterone deficiency is also believed to cause ED in men with abnormally low levels of the hormone. Some men who have come to see me have already been on a testosterone supplementation program. They took regular intramuscular injections or used a patch in order to bring back their libido and erections. Replacement of testosterone in this small group of men—and only in this group—is helpful in overcoming ED.

Finally, there is the dated belief that psychological problems are the fundamental cause for ED. While there are men who do have serious psychological components to their problem, in most there is also a physiological cause. The psychological part is often a response to their ED, manifested as depression or anxiety. Rarely is the situation one where psychological problems are the sole cause of ED.

LIFESTYLE AND ED

While medication and surgery certainly affect ED, nothing makes more of an impact on a man's sexual health than his lifestyle.

There are very particular, modifiable health risks which play major contributory roles in ED. They are obesity, smoking, and excessive drinking. Most often, ED will be the result of a combination of these factors. For instance, if all three risks are part of your health profile you run a greater chance of developing ED. If, however, only one of these components applies to you, your risk is lessened. Each factor seems to join together to intensify the probability of experiencing ED.

Being deficient in one or more of the following components does not automatically mean that you will experience ED. Nevertheless, to a large extent, optimum virility depends on certain lifestyle choices that you make. They include:

- whether or not you smoke
- how much you eat
- how much alcohol you consume
- how much exercise you get
- how you deal with stress
- how much sleep you get
- the quality of your diet
- whether you use harmful drugs

To immediately implement healthy changes that can prevent or help overcome ED, here are the first steps that you can take. All of them will be discussed at length in subsequent chapters as part of my virility-enhancement program. You can begin to take charge of your sexual health right now.

1. Stop Smoking

Of all the behaviors that can damage your health none has been as thoroughly documented as smoking. Not only does it promote heart disease and cancer, but when it is combined with other risk factors, its harmful effects on ED increase dramatically. Consider this:

- Smokers under treatment for heart disease are almost three times as likely to suffer complete ED as nonsmokers.
- Smokers under treatment for hypertension are twice as likely to have complete ED as nonsmokers.
- Smokers with untreated arthritis are more than twice as likely to have complete ED as nonsmokers.

2. Lose Weight

While obesity itself is not a direct cause of ED, being overweight is associated with the deposition of fatty deposits on the interior arterial walls, which in turn is linked to the condition. Unfortunately, Americans, who already lead the world in corpulence, are getting fatter. Studies from the Centers for Disease Control and Prevention indicate that 33 percent of American adults are overweight or obese, up from 25 percent in 1980. Moreover, the rise of this condition among teenagers—21 percent of all twelve- to nineteen-year-olds—continues.

3. Reduce Your Alcohol Intake

For most adults, moderate drinking of beer, wine, or spirits (one to two drinks per day), is not associated with any health or ED risks. But when alcohol is consumed in excess, it acts as a toxic drug with pronounced short- and long-term consequences. Research now links excessive alcohol intake with increased ED. This occurs because alcohol interferes with messages between the brain's pituitary gland and the genitals. Even worse, heavy drinking—more than three drinks per day—is often combined with some variation of the following: steady smoking, overeating, lack of exercise, and drug abuse. This deadly mix nearly always adds to the potential development of ED.

4. Exercise Regularly

The simple equation is this: regular exercise equals better sex. There's a definite connection between being physically active and sustaining an energetic sex life. The converse is true as well: if you don't exercise, you'll be putting a brake on sexual performance.

At the most basic level, it's well known that regular exercise improves overall physical fitness, and that sexual functioning is an important part of that condition. It has been proven that steady exercise:

- improves cardiovascular function, which causes vasocongestion, or raising blood supply to the penis during intercourse, thereby helping to achieve and maintain an erection
- positively affects brain wave activity, which makes you feel energized
- builds stamina, preventing or delaying fatigue during sex
- augments muscle strength, helping to heighten sexual response, a definite asset since orgasm requires considerable muscle activity

- boosts testosterone levels, leading to heightened libido
- decreases percentage of body fat, which can positively alter personal attitudes about sex

5. Reduce the Stress in Your Life

Although more than 80 percent of all ED can be traced to physical causes, there are still some psychological causes to contend with and stress is at the top of the list. Some stress is undeniably good. It's the nonstop, unstinting kind that is perilous to overall well-being. And it has been proven to bring on ED.

6. Get Enough Sleep

Our bodies need sufficient sleep, and this need allows for little, if any, tampering on our part. If you try to deprive yourself of sleep, you will pay a steep price: an impaired ability to have an erection.

Primarily, humans need sleep in order to rejuvenate mentally. Without enough rest, the mind suffers and shows it. Fatigue, difficulty concentrating, forgetfulness, agitation, irritability, and poor decision-making skills are all symptoms. Miss too much sleep and the unpleasant list continues, with dramatic mood shifts, listlessness, and depression. All of these factors have a negative impact on the capability to sustain an erection.

7. Raise Your HDL Levels (the potency aspect of cholesterol no one ever told you about)

Cholesterol is a white, waxy, fatlike substance present in every tissue of the body. Manufactured by the liver from fats, proteins, and carbohydrates, there are two types of cholesterol: low-density lipoprotein (LDL) and high-density lipoprotein (HDL). The high-density variety carries less cholesterol and, as it circulates through the bloodstream, picks up additional cholesterol and takes it back to the liver for excretion. LDL, on the other hand, distributes its load into the blood system and is often referred to as the "bad" cholesterol.

According to the latest research, *total* cholesterol levels in the bloodstream don't seem to affect potency—but the *individual* HDL levels play a powerful role in ED. Men with HDL levels in the high range —greater than 75 mg/dl—rarely have ED. The hope is that men with low HDL levels—less than 35 mg/dl—can raise their levels naturally through diet, exercise, and smoking cessation and subsequently reduce their risk of ED.

8. Lose the Drugs

Cocaine, marijuana, LSD, amphetamines, and barbiturates all have a negative impact on sexual performance, including the capacity to get and keep an erection.

The most amazing fact that I can impart to you about the quest for a successful treatment of ED is this. In the last decade alone the advances in treating this condition have proven to be more significant than all of those made in the last 2,500 years. But even though there is a safe and effective oral treatment for ED, that does not mean that men, and their partners, can now ignore the many other components of good health and satisfying relationships.

A Cure Is Found

As A PHYSICIAN, I am always amazed at the twists and turns of medical science. Contrary to what many people think, medicine is not just about white-coated scientists in sterile laboratories, precise measurements taken by state-of-the-art equipment, and reams of documentation. At its very heart, it's about the thrill of discovery and the pure human intuition that drives researchers to seek answers.

Even so, more than a few of my patients have voiced their displeasure with today's medical researchers, accusing them of hard-heartedness and lack of empathy for the people who need their expertise so badly. This was emphatically stated to me by Fred, a long-time patient in his sixties, whose ED was brought on by his battle with Parkinson's disease.

"Those scientists are more robot than human," he said to me during one visit. "Whenever I see them interviewed on TV they seem so cold and distant. They look like they have no imagination whatsoever."

I immediately disagreed. "Appearances are sometimes deceptive," I told him. "In fact, some of the most far-reaching and important medical discoveries were made by men who made good use of two of the least scientific factors known: timing and luck."

"Really?" Fred asked, skeptically.

"Absolutely. Where life-changing medical discoveries are concerned, a combination of very specific factors is involved. Observation, of course, is key. Attention to how a treatment is working is another. Many times drugs used to treat one condition have positive effects on another illness. But no matter how devoted medical scientists are to their work, timing and luck have often made life-changing detections possible."

"Like what?" Fred asked.

"Like the discovery of some of the most significant breakthroughs in medical history," I told him and cited the invention of the stethoscope by Dr. René Laennec, who observed a group of children scratching a pin on a piece of wood and listening to the resulting noises that could be heard at the other end. Laennec took what he saw and applied it, leading to the now-ubiquitous medical instrument.

Citing another example, I told Fred about the development of the X ray. Working with a glass cathode tube that contained two electrodes, Wilhelm Roentgen observed that a barium-coated screen that was sitting on a nearby bench was glowing with a faint green light. He figured out that some high-speed electron rays had somehow escaped from the cathode tube and penetrated the screen. That observation and further development led to the "pictures" that have saved innumerable lives. And I also mentioned Dr. John Cade, who was using lithium to treat gout in hamsters and noted that the mineral salt immediately calmed them down. Further experimentation proved that it could work for humans, too, and lithium is now an effective treatment for manic-depressive disorders.

Warming up to the subject, I then told Fred that few things could compare to the way that timing and luck paved the way to the discovery of penicillin, which stands as one of the most important and life-saving events in medical history.

Before leaving for a vacation in the summer of 1928, Sir Alexander Fleming inoculated several culture petri dishes with staphylococcal bacteria colonies. Then he stacked the plates on a corner of his laboratory bench and left for his month-long holiday. While he was gone, mold from the mycology laboratory, directly beneath his own, drifted out an open doorway, up the stairwell, and in through the open door of Fleming's lab. They finally settled down on the petri dishes.

As it happened, the temperature in London was unusually cool over the next nine days, which provided perfect growing conditions for the bacterium *Penicillium* to start flourishing in those petri dishes. As the thermometer inched up, Fleming's staph colony, which thrived in a warm environment, started to grow—only to be attacked by the newly formed penicillin. Over the course of Fleming's holiday, the penicillin virtually destroyed the colonies of staphylococcal bacteria.

When Fleming returned he figured out what had happened, and that observation set him on course for future research. Someone leaving a door open, perhaps just an example of forgetfulness, led Fleming to a Nobel Prize for his work in eradicating bacterial illness as a major cause of death.

Fred finally seemed impressed. "If what you say is true," he said, "then maybe someone will get lucky and figure out a way to cure my ED."

The Serendipity Effect

All of the above examples of medical discoveries had a common thread. Each scientist chanced upon a particular circumstance, observed it closely, and because he had an open mind, deduced the more profound implications of what he was seeing. The definition of serendipity is just that: the notion that chance plays an important role in the process of detection. The discovery of a cure for ED was no different. And the path to that discovery began with someone noticing the journey of a molecule of nitric oxide.

Up until a little more than a decade ago, researchers believed that nitric oxide (NO) was basically a harmless food source for bacteria. Then it was discovered that NO was actually an active agent in every part of the body and responsible for many of the cellular changes which continually take place.

For example, in the brain NO helps orchestrate learning and memory. In the immune system, it attacks invading microorganisms. And in the vascular system, it plays a major role in relaxing blood vessels. This last role caught the interest of researchers at the University of California at Los Angeles (UCLA), and it was here that yet another of NO's applications was deduced. While it is well known that erection problems can stem from diabetes, nerve damage, and the side effects of medications, in most cases it's a direct result of poor blood flow through the penis. The UCLA scientists found that when something goes wrong with the NO in penile tissue, blood flow is adversely affected and the result is ED.

As we saw in the last chapter, for an erection to occur, blood not only has to enter the penis, it has to stay there. In a normal flaccid penis, the smooth muscle inside the corpora cavernosa is always contracted. After blood flows in, it immediately flows out again. However, when a man becomes sexually aroused, nerves spark the smooth penile muscle, forcing it to relax. Then the arteries which feed the corpora quickly open up and blood surges into the two spongy chambers of the corpora, expanding them. Then the corpora press onto the veins which normally carry blood from the area. With these exit veins closed tightly, the penis becomes erect.

Just how the nerves actually signal the smooth muscle to relax remained a medical mystery, and this puzzle had impeded progress in finding a cure for ED. After all, if scientists didn't know what prompted the smooth muscle to relax, how could they develop a remedy when it did not? But then chance played a role, once again. One day in 1987, Dr. Jacob Rajfer, a urologist at the UCLA School of Medicine, lost his way in the maze of similar-looking hallways leading to his laboratory and found himself in front of an office with a sign that read: Pharmacology: Smooth Muscle Lab.

As it happened, Dr. Rajfer had been studying ED for quite some time, and had the hunch that erectile problems often occurred when smooth muscle tissue in the corpora cavernosa failed to relax. Unfortunately, at the time, there was little information available about the nature of smooth muscle in the penis. It was known, however, that when viewed under a microscope, it appeared identical to smooth muscle elsewhere in the body.

Dr. Rajfer's timing was fortuitous. Entering the lab and chatting with a researcher, he was informed that, only a week before, Dr. Louis Ignarro, the director of the Smooth Muscle Lab, had finally found the long-sought-after answer to what causes arterial smooth muscle of the body to relax. Dr. Ignarro and his team discovered that when certain neurotransmitters in the blood bind to receptors on the layer of cells lining the insides of arteries (the endothelium), these cells begin to quickly manufacture NO. Moreover, the NO molecule then disperses into the neighboring layer of smooth muscle cells that surround the endothelium, thereby setting off a chemical reaction that makes them relax.

This crucial piece of information was just what Dr. Rajfer was looking for; it logically explained the relaxation of penile tissue. Then he asked a question that took him to the next step toward finding a cure for ED. Since smooth muscle in the corpora cavernosa was also lined with endothelium, wasn't it possible that NO was present and working there as well?

The two doctors decided to team up and try to determine whether or not NO was indeed there, and whether or not it contributed to the erectile process. Using a rabbit for experimentation, they removed strips of tissue from its corpus cavernosa. Then they electrically stimulated the nerves that attached to the smooth muscle in the tissue and, almost immediately, the muscle relaxed. At the same time, the researchers noted a jump in the amount of nitric oxide in the tissue. They then performed similar experiments on both the corpora cavernosa of men with ED and those without it.

Their conclusion: NO is responsible for triggering erections.

THE BRITISH CONNECTION

The next occurrence of timing and luck that was leading researchers ever closer to an oral cure for ED came with the discovery of unexpected and ultimately useful side effects of other medications. In the early 1990s, researchers working in England, at the Sandwich Laboratories of Pfizer Inc., the American-based pharmaceutical company, were delving into gene receptors. Their goal was to find a way to increase blood flow in the body, thereby easing the pain associated with angina pectoris, a prominent symptom of a cardiac condition known as myocardial ischemia. This condition occurs when the heart muscle is deprived of the blood it requires.

As it turned out, the drug they were experimenting with had a very minor impact on the circulation and heart function of the study's volunteers. But as a last effort, the researchers decided to alter the dose regimen to see if it would make any difference. And indeed it did—but not the way the scientists expected it to. UK-92-480 didn't affect blood flow to the chest; it affected blood flow to the penis, resulting in erections.

The Pfizer researchers quickly switched the primary focus of their investigations to the process by which certain enzymes in the body help trigger an erection. The more they experimented with UK-92-480, the code name for the drug that was to be called sildenafil, and later to be given the brand name of Viagra, the more they realized that they had inadvertently stumbled upon something totally new in the annals of medicine. It seemed they discovered a powerful and effective medication for producing erections.

THE NO CONNECTION

Now it was acknowledged that an erection was a multistep chemical process which began with an increase of blood flow through the penile arteries. Nitric oxide, the critical messenger in the muscles, must be present. And, according to the Pfizer researchers, so too must cyclic GMP (guanosine monophosphate), which is the "message" within the muscles that directs them to relax and allow blood to flow.

Sildenafil amplifies this entire process. When it is taken before a romantic encounter, and then followed by sexual stimulation, the entire chemical sequence kicks in without interference. According to Dr. Ian Osterloh, the Pfizer researcher who directed the ensuing sildenafil clinical trials throughout Europe, the drug is an extremely effective inhibitor. What sildenafil does—and does so well—is block a subtype of phosphodiesterase called phosphodiesterase type 5, which is a specific enzyme that hinders the effects of NO. As nature arranged it, this enzyme happens to be in large supply in the penis. Sildenafil prevents the breakdown of cyclic GMP by phosphodiesterase type 5, thereby allowing NO to do its job of relaxing the penile arteries and allowing blood to flow into the corpora cavernosa. And by preventing blood from flowing out of the penis, sildenafil helps provide a firm erection.

The amazing quality of the drug was described by Dr. Osterloh. "In the past," he says, "the major reason we had trouble finding a drug that would cause an erection is that the penis contains blood vessels, sinusoids (the three spongy chambers essential to erection: the two corpora cavernosa and the corpus spongiosum), blood spaces, and smooth muscle cells. But so do a lot of other organs in the body. So, if a man took a drug that caused an erection by dilating blood vessels in the penis, it always caused dilation in other parts of the body as well—many times with some very undesirable side effects."

Finally, with the discovery of sildenafil, there appeared to be a solution for ED that worked specifically where it was needed, and nowhere else in the body.

The next step was to set up clinical trials in order to see just how effective a drug sildenafil was. This was a crucial process because the history of medicine is full of stories about promising medications that worked beautifully on a handful of test subjects. However, when tested scientifically on hundreds of people in double-blind, randomized, two-way, crossover studies, many have failed miserably. Some weren't all that effective. Others produced severe side effects—and sometimes they caused death. At that awful point, the trials would be halted. But with sildenafil there would be dramatically positive results.

THE CLINICAL TRIALS

Testing a potential mass-market drug is no small matter. It takes time, plenty of money, and patience. When a pharmaceutical company believes it has a marketable drug, it must be submitted to rigorous scientific trials. They consist of actual tests on human subjects and can take a decade or more to complete, with time spent to assemble, correlate, and disseminate the data. Pharmaceutical companies estimate that taking a new medication from the research phase through each of the three, sometimes four, individual experimental trials, to the final submission of the data to the Food and Drug Administration costs $500 million on average. For all the time and money spent, the pharmaceutical company is afforded some protection from competitors. Once a drug gets FDA approval, the company then has two decades in which to exclusively produce and sell that drug.

The procedure for drug trials is always the same. Each promising drug starts out with a relatively small Phase I trial in which the new medication is offered to a select group of patients who have not been helped by conventional therapy. This is not without risk: although the drugs have been tested on animals, toxicity to humans is, at this point, unknown. Phase I trials are usually limited to just a dozen or so patients and generally last up to a year.

If the drug appears to be effective and has acceptable side effects, Phase II begins. Now, dozens of people will receive the drug, while dozens more will take placebos (inert substances). At this time, the researchers are looking at the safety and side-effect profile, but they especially want to know if the experimental drug is more effective than both the placebo and any current therapy used to treat the same ailment. If the drug still seems to be working, then Phase III trials start in which hundreds of subjects, some of whom receive the drug, some of whom get a placebo, are used. Neither group, nor the administering physicians, know who is taking which one. Researchers examine the side effects and effectiveness very closely and also seek to determine optimal dosages of the drug. By Phase IV, the drug has been proven to be effective and researchers are fine-tuning the treatment on test subjects, not checking for efficacy, but seeking to determine whether or not any disturbing side effects appear.

Time-consuming as they are, these medical trials are very important. They strive to prove whether the drug works the way researchers claim it will. And they check to make sure that, when dosage recommendations are followed carefully, the patient will be helped. In the end, the overall safety of a drug is a more crucial consideration than its efficacy.

The Viagra Tests

The tests on Viagra (sildenafil) were no different. In the first human trial of the drug, a dozen men in England who were experiencing ED took it three times a day for a week. The results were extremely encouraging but researchers had to pose some realistic questions: Does anyone really want to take a pill three times daily? And who could afford such a costly treatment?

Another short trial was begun. This time, the dozen men took a single dose every day. Remarkably, ten of them showed positive results, and the researchers concluded that the drug was "a well-tolerated and efficacious oral therapy and represents a new class of peripherally acting drugs for the treatment of this condition."

Phase II drug trials spread beyond the west of England to other parts of the United Kingdom, as well as France and Sweden. In one study, forty-two men, between the ages of thirty-four and seventy, all of whom had experienced ED for at least three years, were divided into two groups. Half took Viagra in 25, 50, or 75 mg doses daily while the others received a placebo. Later, the two groups switched pills. After twenty-eight days, more than 90 percent of the men reported significantly improved sexual performance. This was confirmed by the answers they provided on detailed sexual activity questionnaires. Not only were they filled out by the men taking part in the study, they were answered by their partners as well. It turned out that the men who experienced profound improvement had been taking Viagra.

Then a much more extensive study was begun. This time, 351 patients, between the ages of twenty-four and seventy, participated. Randomly, the men were assigned to take the pill at one of three doses (10, 25, or 50 mg) or a placebo. After twenty-eight days, almost 90 percent of the men taking the 50 mg pill reported a threefold improvement in the quality of their sex lives. They cited satisfaction with the frequency, hardness, and duration of their erections.

"The drug has given me back my life," one man told Dr. Osterloh. "It's changed the way I think about myself. I'm a new man," he said.

Viagra had a powerful effect on the men who tried it, and when the Phase II trial ended and the supply of the drug was stopped, there were a lot of complaints and protests from the test subjects. In fact, one test subject, who had developed ED years earlier, pleaded to be allowed to continue using the drug. Viagra, he said, had altered his life. In his case, the researchers relented and gave it to him. He was, after all, almost ninety.

For Phase III, the trials were moved to the United States under the direction of Dr. Tom Lue, a noted San Francisco urologist. Now, unlike the highly successful European trials which had specifically excluded any man whose ED had a physiological basis, the American tests focused solely on men with physical problems. Subjects with atherosclerosis, or a nerve-related problem like diabetes mellitus, were chosen. The results reinforced the power of Viagra. The European trials proved that it could help men whose ED was contributed to by anxiety or emotional problems. Now the American trials showed that ED related to physiological problems could also be overcome.

In the American study, 416 men with ED problems were randomly chosen to receive either a placebo or a 5, 25, 50, or 100 mg daily dose of Viagra over an eight-week period. Once again, when the study was ended a questionnaire was used to assess sexual satisfaction. More than 70 percent of the men answered that 50 mg of Viagra improved their erections. More than 75 percent said that double that dosage imparted the desired effect.

According to Dr. Harin Padma-Nathan, an associate professor in the University of Southern California Department of Urology, who was also a key researcher in the Viagra trials, the drug had far-reaching effects. It was able to specifically target and greatly enhance a man's ability to:

- have an erection
- maintain an erection

- improve orgasm
- enhance the overall quality of sexual intercourse

The American study also addressed the possible side effects of the drug. Every medication has the potential to cause discomfort, sometimes mild, and other times severe. That's why it's always important to ask your doctor about any medication you are about to take. Once in a while, the possible reactions are so off-putting and difficult to live with that a patient will decide to forgo treatment. In the case of the cure for ED, I'm happy to say, that is unlikely to happen.

The potential side effects for men who take Viagra include:

- *Headaches.* They occur in less than 10 percent of subjects.
- *Flushing, or reddening of the face.* This occurs in less than 10 percent of men taking it.
- *Dyspepsia, or gastrointestinal disorder.* Occurs in less than 10 percent of test subjects.
- *Myalgia, or muscle pain.* This is experienced by less than 10 percent of men.
- *Slight alteration in color vision.* This has not been reported in men taking up to 100 mg, in either the American or European trials. However, it has occurred in test doses over 100 mg, which far exceeds the recommended prescription of 50 mg. When it did happen in test subjects, it lasted from several minutes to a few hours. It is not true color blindness, but rather a slight problem in discriminating among blue-green hues.
- *Interaction with other drugs:* Because of adverse side effects, men taking a nitrate-based drug such as sublingual nitroglycerin or isosorbide dinitrate (Isordil) cannot use the drug.

Viagra had much to recommend it, with few, if any, drawbacks, and Dr. Lue presented the results of his study to a packed audience at the annual meeting of the American Urological Society in New Orleans in 1997. "Sildenafil," he told his fellow physicians, "is an effective, well-tolerated oral treatment for patients with ED associated with a broad range of etiologies."

One of the most significant comments about Viagra was made by a leading ED expert whose specialization included psychiatry. "The evidence that Viagra is an effective treatment is overwhelming and ushers in a whole new era," stated Raymond C. Rosen, professor of psychiatry and medicine and co-director of the Center of Sexual and Marital Health, UMDNJ–Robert Wood Johnson Medical School. "It will finally move ED treatment into the realm of primary care medicine. Millions of men will be helped."

At last, a pill for ED had been developed. Quick-acting, virtually side-effect-free, and easy to take, it was the miracle cure men had been hoping for since ED was first known.

A Second Cure Is Found

The development of a second ED oral medication was based on the work of Dr. Adrian Zorgniotti, whose groundbreaking research was discussed in Chapter 2. But if it hadn't been for a fortuitous meeting between Dr. Zorgniotti and Joseph Podolski, the president of Zonagen, a Texas-based pharmaceutical company, his research might never have passed so rapidly from his basement laboratory to a pill that would be marketed worldwide.

In addition to his work with ED patients, Dr. Zorgniotti was a renowned male fertility expert whose work attracted the attention of Joe Podolski and his company. In New York for a meeting, Podolski was shown several new devices that Dr. Zorgniotti had developed to facilitate human reproduction. Unfortunately, Podolski felt that none of them could ever have been brought to market by his company.

However, knowing of Dr. Zorgniotti's creativity and inventiveness, he asked offhandedly as he was preparing to leave if there was anything else he had developed that might be of interest.

The doctor opened his desk drawer and took out a small paper strip and handed it to Podolski. "You might find this intriguing," he said. "I have got a patent on it but it will take me a little while to refine the delivery system."

As Podolski examined the paper, turning it over carefully in his fingers, Dr. Zorgniotti casually detailed that this phentolamine-impregnated strip was capable of restoring erections in men whose erection capabilities had been compromised.

Podolski was stunned. He put down his coat and asked the doctor to fill him in on all his research with phentolamine. By the end of the conversation, it was clear to Podolski that Dr. Zorgniotti, in failing health, had doubts about his own ability to single-handedly realize the full potential of his work. The two men soon agreed to work together to take the drug to the next important level, which would be a fast-acting pill that could be distributed to a much larger market than Dr. Zorgniotti could ever have hoped to reach on his own. "His only concern was that we at Zonagen do justice to his work. This was to be his legacy," said Podolski.

Unfortunately, the Zonagen-Zorgniotti alliance was short-lived because Dr. Zorgniotti died soon after. "We feel that we've honored Adrian's memory with the development of Vasomax," said Podolski. "I wish he had lived to see it."

VASOMAX: THE CLINICAL TRIALS

The basis for Vasomax was Dr. Zorgniotti's original buccal strips, but a fast-dissolving pill was developed soon after. In 1995, this pill was tested with a small group of men in doses of 20, 40, and 60 mg. Blood levels of the drug peaked after thirty minutes following the 20 mg dose, and remained high for two hours after administration of the two higher dosages.

Later, in March 1996, Phase II trials were completed in Germany. In those tests, 160 men were randomly assigned treatment with either 20, 40, or 60 mg of phentolamine, or a placebo. Analysis of the resulting data proved that 40 mg had the best efficacy and safety profile. Interestingly, it also showed that men older than fifty seemed to get the best results. While this was certainly significant clinically, it did not come as a surprise to the researchers. It suggested that the organic causes for ED increase with age, and, therefore, those older than fifty would show impressive restored erectile function.

The only side effect noted by the researchers in this study occurred in the group taking the 40 mg dose. One man reported a stuffy nose. Based on the results of this study, the scientists concluded that a 40 mg dose of Vasomax, in a fast-dissolving tablet, appeared to be an optimally safe and efficient medication for men over fifty.

Phase III trials of Vasomax began immediately in Mexico and were completed by the fall. The study included 148 men at seven centers throughout the country. Men with psychological problems were eliminated but men with primary physical causes of ED were allowed in the study. More than 20 percent of the men had diabetes while 10 percent had undergone prostate surgery. Vasomax showed a 50 percent to 60 percent positive response rate with the men.

In November 1996 additional Phase III studies were conducted in over twenty centers in the United States with 435 men. Men who were receiving cardiovascular therapy as well as those with diabetes were included in the study. They also had to have had a history of ED for at least six months. Men who had radical prostatectomies and spinal cord injuries were intentionally excluded from these trials. This double-blind placebo controlled study showed definite statistical improvement. Men taking the 40 mg Vasomax pill had a 40 percent success rate versus the 17 percent improvement achieved by men taking a placebo.

"What this data tells us," said Raymond Rosen, Ph.D., who reviewed the preliminary data of the Phase III trials and presented his findings at an ED conference in Los Angeles in September 1997, "is that this drug shows definite efficacy in patients with mild to moderate disease, but no efficacy at all for patients with severe ED."

An interesting finding from these studies was that there appeared to be a pronounced race-related improvement in ED. Black men who took 60 mg of Vasomax had a 60 percent improvement at this dose. "Whether this represents something clinically significant," said Dr. Rosen, "or whether blacks are particularly responsive to the drug, is too early to tell."

Dr. Rosen was encouraged by the Vasomax findings. "If you're looking for an on-demand erectogenic agent, Vasomax is close to the perfect formula," he says. "The drug is well tolerated, and with the exception of a stuffy nose, there are no noticeable side effects."

MY WORK WITH VASOMAX

Soon after the results of the Phase III tests were released, I became involved in yet another set of Phase III trials which Zonagen undertook with two thousand men across the United States. In my own experience with the medication, I was able to make some intriguing observations. I found that not all men responded the same way to Vasomax, nor did they all achieve the same results. This made great sense. As individuals, people don't all react to medication the same way. That's one of the reasons why medical science tries to find different ways of treating a malady.

What I did find is that most of the time Vasomax could transform a life devastated by ED. At last, I was able to help my patients with the most effective means available. A fast-acting pill with virtually no side effects produced erections in men who had been incapable of having them, sometimes for a decade or more. The only thing the pill required was normal sexual stimulation. This last point truly distanced Vasomax from the realm of the now-outdated treatments for ED. For the first time, a medication for men tapped into the emotional component of sex.

Remember Frank, the justifiably angry patient who goaded me about finding an oral cure for his ED? He was one of my first patients to try Vasomax. Immediately he was able to achieve the type of natural erection he thought was lost to him forever. With renewed virility and restored confidence, Frank was able to embark on a satisfying long-term relationship.

Frank's story was far from unique. In so many patients I saw the renewal of erections:

- disrupted by atherosclerosis. In the case of Andrew, a fifty-two-year-old with a history of excess weight and high cholesterol, the change was dramatic. Having suffered from ED for five years, his marriage was crumbling as fast as his confidence. As soon as he began taking Vasomax, his life, as he told me, "did a complete 180 degree turn. For the first time in years I feel like myself again. I feel so much better that now I'm even psyched to lose weight and finally get in shape. And I want to give my marriage another try. Now I think we can work things out."
- interrupted for years by diabetes. Harry, a fifty-eight-year-old whose late-developing diabetes had begun to impact on his sex life, had another reaction. "I thought sex was a thing of the past. Between my divorce and my condition, I had actually talked myself into believing that this is the way things have to be. Now that I know they don't have to be that way, it's a whole new world. It's scary—but it's exciting."
- halted by Parkinson's disease. Fred, the one who had given me his opinions of medical research, was another patient who responded incredibly well to Vasomax. While the progression of

his disease was slow, his ED had, effectively, begun to put the brakes on his sex life. His wife of twenty-six years was patient and understanding, but, he admitted, "It just wasn't the same between us. How could it be? With this new drug we're strengthening our bond, and our relationship is growing in a whole new way."

- halted for eighteen months following a serious bicycle injury. Scott, who at twenty-five had experienced some ED, was enormously relieved. "I was beside myself," he told me. "My wife always believed that I would make a full recovery, but I had my doubts. A year and a half without sex is one thing. Thinking that you'll never have it again is another. Now, I'm the man I was—and I can stay that way."

- lapsed due primarily to psychological causes for eight years. While the new medications can eradicate physiologically induced ED in men, we should not forget that it can also be used by men whose problems are psychological in nature. With Edward, a forty-two-year-old who had a history of depression and whose resultant ED made him shy away from women, the change was startling. "I feel better than I ever did," he told me. "I feel that maybe I'm no different from anyone else—for the first time in my life. Thank you for helping me this way."

MY PRACTICE OF SEXUAL MEDICINE

Restoring the optimal sexual health of my male patients doesn't mean that I just prescribe a pill and send them on their way. I regard sexuality as a part of internal medicine, which means that the entire person must be "treated" for optimum, long-lasting results.

The practice of sexual medicine includes finding and matching the correct dosage of a particular medication with an individual patient.

More importantly, it involves seeking out and treating the underlying causes and risk factors for the man's ED. My ongoing support, once treatment has begun, has as its long-term goal:

- sustained success
- prevention of any worsening of the ED
- possible reversal of the damaging effects of ED

I also hope that by taking early aggressive action in those patients who have one or more risk factors for the development of ED, I will be able to help them prevent its onset. That's why I developed my virility-enhancement program, which is described in detail in Chapter 9. The new medications are its cornerstone; the other components build on that solid foundation in a program that can, literally, change your life.

The Miracle Pills at Work

WHENEVER I PRESCRIBE a medication, particularly one that might have to be taken for the rest of a patient's life, I ask the person receiving it a basic question: "Do you wear eyeglasses or contact lenses?" If the answer is yes—as it most often is—I then ask if he would consider living without them. Of course, the answer is always an emphatic No!

I strongly believe in the power of medicine. It can, literally, restore a life altered by illness and pain. In its best use, it can also greatly improve the quality of a life. Today, there is a huge spectrum of medical help available, whether it be cholesterol- or blood-pressure-lowering drugs, insulin to control diabetes, or a host of medicines that keep people alive and able to go on with their lives.

Viagra and Vasomax fit into that category. While some men initially balk at the idea of having to take medicine to help them overcome ED, they soon realize that, like trying to see without eyeglasses, their

THE VIRILITY SOLUTION

lives would be severely compromised without it. The patients who especially welcome the medication are those who have tried the other limited ED options.

This has been the case over and over again with my patients.

ONE MAN'S EXPERIENCE

Ron, a forty-one-year-old electrician, was one of the first men who enrolled in the Phase III Vasomax trials that I supervised. Using two thousand patients from around the country, Zonagen, the manufacturer of Vasomax, began additional research. The participating doctors and subjects knew the drug that was being tested. In this case, it happened to be the 40 mg dose of Vasomax. The goal was to get long-term safety experience with the medication prior to applying to the Food and Drug Administration for formal approval.

"I felt that the sex I was having was just okay," Ron told me on his first visit. "I also knew that it should have been a lot better. I'm not looking for the stamina of a teenager," he admitted, "but now sex doesn't feel the way I know it can be. Getting an erection isn't the problem—it's that I'm not as firm and full as I used to be. Amy, my wife, says it doesn't bother her. But I'm very aware of it—and it upsets me. A lot."

Ron was so dismayed by his problem that he mentioned it to his family physician after a routine checkup. His results were fine, with the exception of an elevated cholesterol count. At 260 milliliters per deciliter (ml/dl) it was high, and his doctor told him that he should work on lowering it to a healthier level of under 200 ml/dl.

When Ron voiced his sexual concerns, he was stunned by the doctor's reaction. "You're in your forties. What do you expect?" he was told. "You have to expect a little letdown in your sexual performance as you age. It's just the way it is."

Not for Ron it wasn't. Dissatisfied with both his doctor's interpretation of, and insensitivity to, his problem, he made an appointment with a urologist for more detailed testing. Maybe, he thought, his doctor had missed a clue that would solve his ED.

After providing a complete medical history and answering questions about masturbation, morning erections, and his libido, Ron underwent a more complex physical exam which included the health of his genitals and prostate gland. Then he had to undergo what he referred to as "the single most embarrassing event of my adult life."

The doctor explained to him that in order to fully determine the extent of Ron's ED, he would begin tests to measure and scrutinize erectile function. Standing naked in front of the doctor, Ron saw what was going to happen next. The urologist was approaching him with an ultra-thin needle and his aim was low. Extremely needle-phobic, Ron tried to calm himself while he was injected in the base of his penis with tri-mix, the combination of papaverine, phentolamine, and prostaglandin E-1.

Within five minutes, the drugs began to take effect, resulting in an erection. But Ron's experience wasn't about to end there. Left alone in the examining room, he was instructed to remain standing and masturbate. Erotic materials were provided in the event that he needed them. Then, in order to test the effectiveness of the tri-mix, the doctor had to know whether or not he had successfully masturbated and how long his erection lasted. To ascertain this information, he checked on Ron every ten minutes to note penis rigidity and fullness. For almost twenty minutes after the injection, his erection was still hard, then began to subside. Needless to say, nothing about this episode even vaguely approached normal sexual response.

Nevertheless, comparing the test results with his medical history, the urologist was able to diagnose a mild blood flow disruption to the penis. He believed that Ron's erection problem was triggered by early arteriosclerosis, or hardening of the arteries. This, the doctor informed him, was most likely linked to his elevated cholesterol. That, in turn, was connected to arterial blockage, which resulted in his mild blood flow problem.

Ron left the doctor's office feeling, as he later put it, "about as lousy as I've ever felt. Telling me to inject myself every time I wanted to have sex with my wife was not what I wanted to hear. I had to find another way."

THE BEGINNING OF A NEW LIFE

At the suggestion of a friend who was already participating in the Vasomax study, Ron came to see me. After carefully screening him, I concurred with the urologist. For the most part, his health was excellent. He didn't smoke, and exhibited no signs of hypertension, diabetes, prostate cancer, or Parkinson's disease, the major ailments typically associated with ED.

I told Ron that his primary symptoms, which included slower arousal time, the need for increased stimulation to achieve an erection, and the inability to maintain an erection, were early signs of ED. He was accepted into the study and before he left that afternoon, I gave him a one-month supply of Vasomax pills, along with diaries that both he and his wife were to fill in as soon as a sexual encounter was over. I told him that a stuffy nose was a possible side effect, and that he might feel lightheaded or a quickening pulse. He should carefully record any unusual changes he might experience.

Before he left, Ron asked me one more question: "If the pills work for me, will I have to take them forever?"

I told him what I tell all my patients taking the new medications. Reactions vary from patient to patient, depending on the nature of their particular erectile problems. But if it turned out that Ron did need them indefinitely, I didn't foresee a problem. "Look at it this way," I said. "The help you need is available to you. Just take that little white pill—and live the most satisfying life you can."

Like so many men whom I've treated, Ron now regards his sex life as pre- and post-Vasomax. In the old era, he and his wife would try to have sex once or twice a week, with a lot of uncertainty on Ron's part. Post-Vasomax, they quickly rediscovered the joys of spontaneous sex. Ron's fear of inadequacy vanished. And gone forever was the very unpleasant option of having to inject himself.

Ron summed up his experience in a way I'll always remember. "When I left your office after taking Vasomax for the first time, Amy and I went to dinner. I started to feel differently. I became acutely aware of how lovely she looked, and, all of a sudden, my emotional response to her was matched by a really powerful physical urge. I was overcome with desire for her. In fact, we skipped dessert in the restaurant—and had it at home, if you know what I mean."

THE ROMANCE PILL

I certainly did. Unlike the vacuum penis pump or the injection of the tri-mixture into the penis, the ED medications are able to tap into the emotional experience of sex. The pump is a machine. It gets the job done, but it doesn't require that the man using it have any erotic or romantic involvement with his partner. The same is true for tri-mix. The fact that these two treatments lack an emotional connection has been a source of steady complaint from the partners of the patients who use them.

It's a difficult situation. It's as though the pre-erection mental stress and insecurity suffered by the man with ED transfer to his partner once he has achieved his goal. I've often heard it said by those partners that "Now that he can perform, I wonder whether he's just going through the motions because he can have sex, or whether he really cares about me."

With Viagra and Vasomax there is never any doubt. The fact is that without desire and erotic stimulation, the drugs won't work; they're not aphrodisiacs. These amazing medications restore the natural sequence of events that is unique to each couple. Without doubt, they are the closest thing I have seen to normal erectile function.

Here's what Ron and Amy recorded in their post-sex diaries:

Ron's entry reported that "I can't remember the last time we were out for a drive and then suddenly pulled over to a shady spot so that we could climb into the back seat. Of course, neither of us is seventeen, so maneuvering took a bit of doing. But you know what? We laughed, and that made the level of excitement reach an even higher peak. The idea that I didn't have to worry about the possibility of failure has made every encounter that much better. It's like we're climbing a sexual ladder and every rung is stronger than the one before."

Amy's diary said that "I'm amazed. Speechless and amazed. I haven't seen Ron this happy and confident in a long, long time. As for me—I'm just reaping the rewards of this wonderful pill. We're closer than ever. Thank you so much."

Other participants wrote of similar experiences. "I'm just delighted with the results," said Marcia, whose husband, Steve, had suffered with ED for eight of their twenty-two married years. "In the past, lots of times sex was less a pleasure and more an ordeal. We'd talk, strategize, and plan; you'd think we were storming the Normandy beaches. Now, Steve can take his time and concentrate on the romance of the moment. I'm thrilled; it's such a turn-on."

Steve, who at forty-nine has type I diabetes, which requires daily insulin injections, had had a terrible time dealing with his ED. "But now I view the pill as a way to express my love for my wife, who has been so incredibly supportive and loving all these years. We can have extended sex that goes on longer than it ever did—even before my illness. I can hold off and maintain or even regain an erection. The medication has returned something precious to us that I thought was lost forever."

Harvey, a fifty-one-year-old pizza shop owner, had another reaction. "It's better if I haven't eaten a big meal. After taking the pill, the slightest sexual stimulation within half an hour sets me off. I get an erection that lasts a long time. Usually, I go to bed late but sometimes I wake up with a powerful erection and Estelle and I do it again."

Estelle concurred. "I can't believe this wonderful episode in our lives. The best thing is that Harv doesn't feel rushed—which I just love."

My Goal in Prescribing the Drugs

Helping my patients regain a quality of life that involves their ability to function sexually is the objective of my treatment. Without a doubt, the pills, along with my virility-enhancement program, are now the best ways for overcoming ED. I've found that the most suitable candidates for the pills are those who are in reasonably good health, without any unstable or acute illness. These are the men who are ready, willing, and able to do everything possible to enhance their chances for success.

Frequently in medicine there are multiple treatments available for a single ailment. For example, each day I need to decide which of the fifteen different blood pressure medications I will prescribe for a patient or which of the many antibiotics should be used to treat pneumonia. My decision is based on clinical experience, severity of the disease, side-effect profile of the medication, and unfortunately, at times, the cost of the medication.

With ED, the same decision-making process is required. I use Vasomax for those men who clearly have psychological and early mild erectile dysfunction. Because of its safety profile, I might attempt its use in a more severely impaired person by raising the dosage from the typical 40 mg level to a higher 80 mg, observing for blood pressure and cardiac changes. I have found the response—or lack of—to Vasomax to be a clue to the severity of the patient's underlying nerve and blood vessel disease. For example, those men with more advanced atherosclerosis or diabetes typically will not respond to Vasomax at its highest (80 mg) dose.

I believe Viagra is a more powerful and effective medication. Urologists involved in the studies have described its effectiveness in patients with moderate to severe ED and even in men who have failed tri-mix injection therapy. Viagra has also proven effective for patients for overcoming the ED effects of various medications that they require. Viagra is a new prescription agent and a larger body of clinical data will be needed before we truly understand all of its applications. Trials will soon be underway to study the effects of the drug in patients who are at high risk for ED. These include men undergoing radical prostate surgery as well as those men with diabetes who are still functioning but are expected to develop ED in the future. This prophylactic use of Viagra may ultimately result in enhanced oxygenation, and therefore improved penile health.

I am confident that doses of up to 100 mg of Viagra can be used to satisfy most couple's needs. However, as with most medications, we should always use the lowest effective dosage in order to reduce possible side effects. The drug is fast-acting, according to Pfizer's Dr. Ian Osterloh. "When taken on an empty stomach, many men in the study were able to have sexual intercourse within twenty minutes."

My experience with Vasomax has suggested that the pills can be taken at least ten times a month without any side effects. I have advised the men in my study to use it no more than once daily. Vasomax facilitates erections for at least ninety minutes after taking the pill. However, after taking a standard 40 mg dose, some of my patients have reported achieving a second erection with sexual stimulation hours later without any additional medication.

But before I even think of prescribing the medications, I first take a complete medical history to determine whether there are any major underlying problems that are producing ED. I inquire about diet and exercise programs, too. I'm particularly interested if a patient is an avid cyclist. It now appears that the constant pounding in the genital area, which bicyclists routinely absorb, can cause a deterioration of the blood flow in the delicate penile arteries.

I ask as well if the patient has an already-diagnosed medical disorder, such as diabetes, arthritis, hypothyroidism, or hypertension, which can have an impact on their condition. If any of these problems are present, I explain that I will treat both the medical disorder as well as the resultant ED. Finally, I perform a complete medical work-up, including blood tests and blood pressure test.

Sometimes, a man won't have a specific illness associated with ED, or have suffered an injury. His cholesterol is normal and there is no obvious reason for his problem. Unlike other medical problems, the actual cause of ED is not a determinant in its treatment. I believe protracted testing to pinpoint the physical or psychological underlying causes of ED isn't necessary at the outset. What is important is the restoration of erectile function. Letting this problem go untreated will only lead to potentially harmful repercussions in the man's personal life.

Oftentimes, over the course of treatment, clues begin to surface about the exact nature of the problem. Whenever possible, I will follow these up and work toward a specific diagnosis. Sometimes minor adjustments in lifestyle, and dietary and exercise modifications are all that it takes to halt the progression of ED.

I tell my patients that, in some cases, ED is an ailment that will require continual treatment that we will overcome together. But by following the treatments outlined in this book, they can expect changes that will, eventually, result in sexual satisfaction for themselves and their partners. In some cases, special psychological counseling may be required to help mend the anxiety or anger that is often ED-related.

Two Patients' Stories

There are a variety of medical histories that make a man a candidate for the drugs. Consider these two patients who coped with their ED problems in different ways. Still, I decided that both would get good results from Vasomax.

When Bill, a thirty-six-year-old video store owner, enrolled in the Vasomax study, he thought his sex life as he knew it was over. He complained to me of persistent "unsatisfactory" erections. "Everything was fine," he related, "until my accident. I've been playing pickup basketball games since I was in high school and I've had my share of minor injuries, just like everyone else. But then, one Sunday, there was a chain reaction fall and some guy inadvertently kicked me in the scrotum. Ever since then my sexual performance has been extremely unreliable. I've lost my fiancée and I don't want to lose the ability to have normal sex for the rest of my life.

"One doctor I went to suggested an implant. That's extreme, since I was having some erections—and besides, I feel I'm much too young for that. And forget about the shots. To me, injections are a dire-emergency fallback position. I tried the natural route, too, everything from a macrobiotic diet to high colonics. Then there was acupuncture. I even tried that plastic vacuum pump. You know what happened with that? I met a really attractive woman at a friend's wedding and we hit it off. After several dates we thought that it was time for the relationship to progress. I really liked her, you know? So I went into the bathroom and used the pump, and came out with that rubber constriction ring on the base of my penis that helps keep it hard. She took a look and I guess she was kind of shocked. She said, 'I never thought I'd be doing it with a bionic man.' And that was the end of that relationship.

"So I've been living the private life of a monk. You're my last resort. Please—my whole life is ahead of me."

Bill's ED was physically induced and psychologically intensified; tests confirmed his own diagnosis. He wanted to get help and remained hopeful that his situation could be corrected. The 40 mg dose of Vasomax was the help he was looking for. "I can't begin to tell you how great this is," he told me a month later. "I feel like I'm back in the world again, that I'm allowed to be attracted to women and have fulfilling sex, if I want to, when I want to. I *knew* there would be a cure—I'm just so relieved that it came along in my lifetime."

Another patient who sought to enroll in the study was John, a fifty-eight-year-old maintenance crew supervisor who had recently undergone triple bypass surgery. For the five years prior to the operation, his heart disease had put a brake on his sexual relationship with Harriet, his wife. What was frustrating to both of them was that now that his heart was repaired, he still had ED. Harriet, who accompanied John to my office, put it this way: "We thought that the surgery would put the bad times behind us, that the pressures and stress of his illness would be gone. When we finally felt the time was right, John couldn't respond, no matter what I tried. We both were disappointed. And, I'll tell you the truth, I was a little angry, too. I want to be supportive and reassuring, but I'm having a really hard time. We fight a lot. I feel like no matter what medicine has to offer, nothing will help us."

I wasn't surprised to hear Harriet's view. Being the partner of a man with ED is no easy matter. Many couples maintain a truce; either they won't talk about the problem or they ignore it in the false belief that it doesn't exist. Sadly, their self-induced silence not only distances them physically, but emotionally as well. Often, the relationship, already on shaky ground, disintegrates completely. And ED can foster doubt in the partner, as well.

As Harriet said, "I thought I knew what the trouble was after the operation. John just didn't find me attractive anymore. After all, we've been married for twenty-five years and I've had three children. I don't look like I did when we first got married. I thought that now that he had recovered his health, he wanted a younger, more vibrant woman at his side. On one level I was devastated but ironically, on another, I was kind of relieved. Now I wouldn't have to feel rejected because we didn't have to try to have sex. I looked elsewhere for comfort, and buried myself—like so many unhappy people do—in my work."

John looked stunned as Harriet told her side of the ED story. "I never felt that way," he said to her. "I thought you'd leave me because I was failing you."

After consulting John's cardiologist, I was able to reduce the dosage of some of his heart medications, which I felt were contributing to his erection problems. I also enrolled the couple in the Vasomax study.

While the 40 mg of Vasomax did them both a world of good, it was the foundation on which they could start to rebuild their torn relationship. John, who was so beaten down by years of erectile failure, needed to face the profound psychological damage that both he and Harriet had experienced. Harriet, in turn, could benefit by facing her anger and doubts. I suggested to them that they seek professional help. Happily, they took my advice and began seeing a therapist who specialized in marital issues.

THE DOSAGES: WHAT THEY MEAN

Before I provide a man with the ED medications, I have a serious discussion with him about the importance of understanding how the pills work. I make it very clear that the erection pill will allow him to function sexually within a relatively large window of opportunity. It does not, however, mean that the medications can cure the condition that caused ED in the first place. I also reiterate that more is not better. Doubling a dose will not make a better lover. In fact, it might bring on some undesirable side effects, such as plummeting blood pressure, light-headedness, and a racing heart.

THE POTENTIAL SIDE EFFECTS

Viagra is prescribed in standard 50 mg doses and is taken no more than an hour before an encounter. If you have a more severe case of ED, your doctor may recommend a higher dose. Viagra has been reported to cause very mild headaches. Other possible side effects can include facial flushing or gastrointestinal disturbances, minor problems that quickly subside. In addition, it should be noted that Viagra cannot be used if you're taking nitrate-based drugs, because of adverse side effects.

In my trials with Vasomax, men took the lowest available dose, 40 mg, thirty minutes before an anticipated sexual encounter. For men with more advanced ED, the dose was increased to 80 mg. Although Vasomax can produce side effects, the one that has been most commonly reported—a stuffy nose—subsides within an hour.

I tell the patient to contact me immediately if he is suffering any severe or unusual reaction to the medication. One person may be more sensitive to a drug than others. Informing me if anything amiss occurs allows me to make adjustments in the dosage at once. For most men, however, there are no unusual or serious side effects. These medications are stable, fast-acting, and directed specifically to the penis. As I have seen many times, as soon as a patient becomes physiologically adjusted to the drugs, his concerns about side effects evaporate. For him, it's just like taking an aspirin.

WHEN A PATIENT DOESN'T WANT MEDICATION

For some people, the idea of having to take medication is less than thrilling. It signifies getting older, losing control of their bodies, and facing their mortality. Even though the ED drugs have proven to be so successful, some of my patients are still reluctant to use them. Or they use them for a while and suddenly stop. I think this is linked to the unspoken desire to feel "normal" and in control. But if a patient stops taking the drugs, thinking that he is cured permanently, he is going to subject himself to another, potentially more devastating round of failure, deflated self-confidence, and embarrassment.

Using ED medication is hardly a sign of weakness or inadequacy. On the contrary, taking it means that a man is dealing with his problem and, in fact, overcoming it in the most painless, practical way possible. *It basically comes down to this: Without the drugs, function is going to remain impaired. With them, it will be corrected.*

ADVANCES IN SEXUAL MEDICINE

One of the most exciting aspects of my work in sexual medicine is seeing the far-reaching potential of the new drugs. Restoring virility to those who have suffered, along with their partners, for so long is nothing less than exhilarating. I have seen lives reclaimed, revitalized, and virtually transformed. Relationships strained to their limits have not only been repaired; they've been strengthened, too. I've been witness to the rejuvenating effects of sex in those who were denied its pleasures for far too long.

We're in a whole new era of sexual medicine, where, thankfully, many men are coming forward and voicing their desire to be helped. What counts most is the person's commitment to addressing his condition and following all of the steps necessary to achieve success. Naturally, each man responds uniquely to the medications, but I have noted some consistent patterns in the men who take them. For instance:

- self-esteem is elevated
- relationships are solidified
- in some cases, unfulfilling commitments are severed once virility is restored
- stress and anxiety diminish
- a sense of wholeness, along with an integration of mind and body, takes place
- a newfound confidence spills over to other areas of life
- for those without partners, there is a renewed willingness to seek companionship
- for some, it offers the same freedom to seek and enjoy the pleasure they knew as teenagers
- for others, the liberating effects allow for a total exploration of the very nature of their sexuality—and some real surprises

Because so many men are coming forward and voicing their need for this restoration to what it used to be, let's take a look at how this process actually occurs.

The First Step to a Renewed Sex Life

As you've already seen, medical science now knows that, most often, ED has a physical cause. Acknowledging that breakthrough takes us— physicians and patients alike—into the new world of sexual medicine. Today, the physiological aspects of ED can be treated. But without looking at and addressing another crucial component of a man's sex life, the medications will take that man only so far. Facing the psychological reverberations that ED causes in men and their partners is an equally important part of treating the condition successfully. Dealing with the aftereffects of a renewed sex life is another.

Sex involves two people, and their feelings must be recognized. I know many men shy away from talking about their ED for a number of reasons, including embarrassment, frustration, and fear. But without facing the problem, in all its complexity, it can't be solved to the mutual satisfaction of both partners. In order to fully overcome ED and its far-reaching repercussions in a couple, several actions need to be taken:

- First of all, a man must acknowledge his problem and talk to his partner about it.
- Second, he needs to discuss the treatment options with his doctor.
- Third—and possibly most important of all—he has to ask himself what sex, both physically and emotionally, means to him.

As I've stated throughout this book, without an emotional connection to your sexual partner, the pills alone won't give you the deep, satisfying awareness that defines great sex. For those of you who took your sex lives for granted until it changed, this is a golden opportunity. Not only do you have available the means to restore your sexual function; now you can bring new emotional perspective to your relationship, giving it a stronger, more resilient bond that will enhance your sexual experiences as well as those of your partner.

The long-reaching effects of the ED medications will take men and their partners into a new phase of their lives. I would be remiss if I didn't guide you through this uncharted territory. To do that, we have to take the first step toward the resolution of ED. And that means that the problem has to be faced. There is a painless and quick method that can help you do that. All you have to do is take the time to answer fifteen questions.

A Unique Test

I've found the International Index of Erectile Function, or IIEF, to be an extremely valuable tool. Its questions provide an exceptionally effective method to measure the extent of ED. Developed by six ED experts, the IIEF has been translated into more than twenty languages and is used worldwide. Dr. Raymond Rosen, a member of the team, says, "The beauty of the IIEF is that it is specifically designed to assess a man's current level of erectile dysfunction. It precisely gets answers in five key domains: erectile function, sexual desire, orgasmic function, intercourse satisfaction, and overall gratification."

I used the IIEF with every patient in my clinical trials. Extremely helpful, it gave the men an objective evaluation of their current level of ED. You now have the opportunity in the privacy of your home to take the same test to determine your ED level. To be honest and fair to yourself, as well as your partner, answer these questions truthfully. No one is looking over your shoulder and the object of the questionnaire is not to "pass" or "fail." Rather, its function is to give you the answers you need to obtain the best solution to your problem.

After filling in the appropriate boxes, rate yourself with the accompanying scale. The IIEF will allow you to identify the key areas in which you may have ED problems. The answers will indicate whether you should follow up the quiz with a visit to your physician. Also keep in mind that the following definitions should be applied when you consider your answers:

- "Sexual activity" includes caressing, foreplay, masturbation, and intercourse.
- "Sexual intercourse" is defined as penetration of your partner.
- "Sexual stimulation" includes situations like foreplay, looking at erotic pictures, or viewing an X-rated video.
- "Ejaculate" is the ejection of semen from the penis or the feeling that it is taking place.

If you decide to see your doctor and you opt for an oral medication to treat your ED, you can chart your progress by retaking the quiz over the subsequent months. Chances are good that, after taking oral medication, following my virility-enhancement program, and working on your relationship with your partner, your answers will be quite different just a month later. (Photocopy these pages so that you'll have a handy copy of the quiz when you want to retest yourself.)

The IIEF Questionnaire

NOTE: For each question, please check one box only.

The first five questions refer to erectile function.

1. Over the last month, how often were you able to get an erection during sexual activity?

   - ❑ 0   No sexual activity
   - ❑ 5   Almost always or always
   - ❑ 4   Most times (much more than half the time)
   - ❑ 3   Sometimes (about half the time)
   - ❑ 2   A few times (much less than half the time)
   - ❑ 1   Almost never or never

2. Over the last month, when you had erections with sexual stimulation, how often were your erections hard enough for penetration?

   - ❑ 0   No sexual activity
   - ❑ 5   Almost always or always
   - ❑ 4   Most times (much more than half the time)
   - ❑ 3   Sometimes (about half the time)
   - ❑ 2   A few times (much less than half the time)
   - ❑ 1   Almost never or never

3. Over the last month, when you attempted intercourse, how often were you able to penetrate (enter) your partner?

- ❏ 0 Did not attempt intercourse
- ❏ 5 Almost always or always
- ❏ 4 Most times (much more than half the time)
- ❏ 3 Sometimes (about half the time)
- ❏ 2 A few times (much less than half the time)
- ❏ 1 Almost never or never

4. Over the last month, during sexual intercourse, how often were you able to maintain your erection after you had penetrated (entered) your partner?

- ❏ 0 Did not attempt intercourse
- ❏ 5 Almost always or always
- ❏ 4 Most times (much more than half the time)
- ❏ 3 Sometimes (about half the time)
- ❏ 2 A few times (much less than half the time)
- ❏ 1 Almost never or never

5. Over the last month, during sexual intercourse, how difficult was it to maintain your erection to completion of intercourse?

- ❏ 0 Did not attempt intercourse
- ❏ 1 Extremely difficult
- ❏ 2 Very difficult
- ❏ 3 Difficult
- ❏ 4 Slightly difficult
- ❏ 5 Not difficult

STEVEN LAMM, M.D.

The next three questions refer to satisfaction with intercourse.

6. Over the last month, how many times have you attempted sexual intercourse?

❑ 0   No attempts
❑ 1   1–2 attempts
❑ 2   3–4 attempts
❑ 3   5–6 attempts
❑ 4   7–10 attempts
❑ 5   11–20 attempts

7. Over the last month, when you attempted sexual intercourse how often was it satisfactory to *you*?

❑ 0   Did not attempt intercourse
❑ 5   Almost always or always
❑ 4   Most times (much more than half the time)
❑ 3   Sometimes (about half the time)
❑ 2   A few times (much less than half the time)
❑ 1   Almost never or never

8. Over the last month, how much have you enjoyed sexual intercourse?

❑ 0   No intercourse
❑ 5   Very highly enjoyable
❑ 4   Highly enjoyable
❑ 3   Fairly enjoyable
❑ 2   Not very enjoyable
❑ 1   No enjoyment

The next two questions refer to orgasmic function.

9. Over the last month, when you had sexual stimulation or intercourse, how often did you ejaculate?

   ❏ 0   No sexual stimulation/intercourse
   ❏ 5   Almost always or always
   ❏ 4   Most times (much more than half the time)
   ❏ 3   Sometimes (about half the time)
   ❏ 2   A few times (much less than half the time)
   ❏ 1   Almost never or never

10. Over the last month, when you had sexual stimulation or intercourse how often did you have the feeling of orgasm (with or without ejaculations)?

   ❏ 0   No sexual stimulation/intercourse
   ❏ 5   Almost always or always
   ❏ 4   Most times (much more than half the time)
   ❏ 3   Sometimes (about half the time)
   ❏ 2   A few times (much less than half the time)
   ❏ 1   Almost never or never

The next two questions ask about sexual desire. In this context, sexual desire is defined as a feeling that may include wanting to have a sexual experience (for example, masturbation or intercourse), thinking about having sex, or feeling frustrated due to lack of sex.

11. Over the last month, how often have you felt sexual desire?

   ❏ 5   Almost always or always
   ❏ 4   Most times (much more than half the time)

❑ 3 Sometimes (about half the time)

❑ 2 A few times (much less than half the time)

❑ 1 Almost never or never

12. Over the last month, how would you rate your level of sexual desire?

❑ 5 Very high

❑ 4 High

❑ 3 Moderate

❑ 2 Low

❑ 1 Very low or none at all

The next two questions refer to overall sexual satisfaction.

13. Over the last month, how satisfied have you been with your overall sex life?

❑ 5 Very satisfied

❑ 4 Moderately satisfied

❑ 3 About equally satisfied and dissatisfied

❑ 2 Moderately dissatisfied

❑ 1 Very dissatisfied

14. Over the last month, how satisfied have you been with your sexual relationship with your partner?

❑ 5 Very satisfied

❑ 4 Moderately satisfied

❑ 3 About equally satisfied and dissatisfied

❑ 2 Moderately dissatisfied

❑ 1 Very dissatisfied

The last question refers, once again, to erectile function.

15. Over the last month, how do you rate your confidence that you can get and keep your erection?

   ❏ 5 Very high
   ❏ 4 High
   ❏ 3 Moderate
   ❏ 2 Low
   ❏ 1 Very low

What the Scores Mean

All the queries break down into five specific areas, or domains, as follows. Add your scores to the appropriate column on the right.

Domain	Questions	Score Range	Maximum Score	Your Score
Erectile Function	1, 2, 3, 4, 5, 15	0–5	30	
Orgasmic Function	9, 10	0–5	10	
Sexual Desire	11, 12	1–5	10	
Intercourse Satisfaction	6, 7, 8	0–5	15	
Overall Satisfaction	13, 14	1–5	10	

Once you have your numbers down, use the following interpretations to determine how mild or severe your ED is.

Erectile function. In most cases, ED is a steadily worsening condition that can be slowed down, and in some cases reversed, through the use of oral medication. If your answers to questions 1, 2, 3, 4, 5, and 15 add up to 24 or less, then drug intervention may be a viable solution for you. If your responses fall into this range, I suggest that you make an appointment with your doctor, take the questionnaire with you, and discuss the possibility of beginning a course of oral ED medication. Vasomax is generally effective for men with scores between 13 and 24 while Viagra can treat the entire spectrum of dysfunction.

Score	Interpretation of ED
0–6	Severe
7–12	Moderate
13–18	Mild to moderate
19–24	Mild
25–30	None

Orgasmic function. Ejaculation with a semi-erect or soft penis is a strong indicator that you have a penile problem that is physical. If you scored between 0 and 8 in this domain, drug intervention may be needed. Consult with your physician about the right medication for you.

Score	Interpretation of ED
0–2	Severe
3–4	Moderate
5–6	Mild to moderate

7–8	Mild
9–10	None

Sexual desire. Lack of desire for sex is a complex issue. It can be brought on by any number of physical or psychological problems, ranging from testosterone deficiencies, medications for depression, to cardiovascular disease, high blood pressure, and diabetes, to stress, anger, or frustration. As is always the case with illness, whether it has a psychological or physical cause, consulting with your physician is the best place to start treatment.

Score	Interpretation of ED
0–2	Severe
3–4	Moderate
5–6	Mild to Moderate
7–8	Mild
9–10	None

Intercourse satisfaction. This domain specifically covers a man's ability to achieve satisfactory penetration of his partner. Almost universally, a lower score is linked to a higher degree of erectile difficulty. If your score in this domain is between 0 and 12, drug intervention may be needed.

Score	Interpretation of ED
0–3	Severe
4–6	Moderate
7–9	Mild to moderate
10–12	Moderate
13–15	None

Overall satisfaction. How a man adjusts psychologically to a decrease, or loss, of sexual function is often a reflection of the level of intimacy and support he shares with his partner. If you score low in this domain, I recommend that you and your partner read the next chapter to determine what you can do to restore the intimacy that produces the greatest satisfaction in a relationship.

Score	Interpretation of ED
0–2	Severe
3–4	Moderate
5–6	Mild to moderate
7–8	Mild
9–10	None

THE NEXT STEP

Answering the questionnaire and assessing your numbers will give you an honest indication of the extent of your ED. But keep in mind that while the IIEF is an enormously helpful aid, it should not be used as a sole means of diagnosis. Most importantly, it should not replace a visit to your doctor. Use the IIEF as a supporting document when you see him. With answers in hand, it will be easier for you to approach your physician for help. And, in turn, it will simplify treatment options for the doctor as well.

Taking the test is a big step toward dealing with your ED. Knowing the extent of your problem can lead you to its solution. But before you make that doctor's appointment, think about another person you need to speak to—your partner. Remember, you are not the only person whose life is being affected dramatically by ED. Your partner is involved, too, and deserves to know what is going on. Continued silence will only serve to further erode what may have become a rocky relationship for a very long period of time. Ending that bumpy period can have enormous implications for both of you.

Whether it's a precious commodity that is enjoyed often or a dark subject hidden away in the closets of a troubled marriage, where sex is placed within a relationship says a lot about the two people involved. But no matter how open or closed the connection is, it is fraught with intense feelings.

The new sexual medications have the power to instantly change your relationship because the drugs bring, in their wake, a whole new area of emotional response based on the feelings of a couple. Whether they are married or living together, dating frequently or seeing each other once in a while, whether they are straight or gay, the same basic rule applies. If the core connection between two people is strong, then they can build on it, creating a reinforced bridge that will take them to more intimate places. If, however, there has been anger and frustration, suddenly having a restored sex life can be, at the very least, unsettling.

Either way, the psychological implications for a couple whose lives have been affected by ED must be addressed. And beyond that, a revitalized world of intimacy exists for those who want it.

The Road to Heightened Intimacy

TAKING A PILL to regain lost erectile function is an incredible development in the history of drug intervention. But the pill itself cannot obliterate the other problems a couple experiencing ED may have. In fact, in certain circumstances, it may even add to the existing issues with which the pair has had to cope.

One of my greatest concerns as a physician is that the new treatment for ED gives people an unrealistic expectation about their ability to immediately cure their emotional relationships along with their physical ones.

Nothing could be further from the truth.

It is no secret that men and women react differently to sex— before, during, and after it takes place. The availability of a new quick, painless treatment for ED can have one impact on men and quite another on women. Consider the comments I've heard in my office:

From a thirty-three-year-old man under tremendous work-related stress: "The pill is the best thing that could have happened to me."

The comments of his partner, a twenty-nine-year-old lawyer who was equally busy: "Right now we can have the sex we want when time allows for it—which isn't very often."

From a fifty-two-year-old man whose extra poundage and drinking made ED a constant companion: "In one way I feel great because I can have sex again. But in another I feel awful, because I can't hide behind my weight anymore."

His fifty-four-year-old wife had a different view of the situation: "For the last five years his primary relationship has been with food. Now everything has changed and, frankly, I'm not happy about it. It sort of puts the focus on me now."

A forty-six-year-old man, on the verge of a divorce after eight years of marriage, told me: "Ever since I found out that a drug could help me, I've wondered how to use it. Our marriage was based, to a large degree, on sex. For two years we've been trying to find other ways to communicate. We never did. Having the means to have sex again is wonderful—but I have to ask myself, what kind of relationship did we have in the first place?"

His forty-three-year-old wife concurred: "He's right. It was a big reality check to see how little we had in common. Yes—I'd like to have sex with him again. But where do we go from there?"

THE SPEED AGE

It's not surprising that the remarks I hear range from fearful to ecstatic. A profound change in one's sexual habits is no small matter, and cannot be dealt with in the time it takes to swallow a little pill.

Time, in a variety of ways, is an important issue where ED and its implications—as well as treatment—are concerned. Unfortunately, in today's society, we're used to quick fixes. In fact, we have come to anticipate that the time it takes to accomplish something will continually be shortened.

Think about it. We expect our computers to find and disseminate information at a nanosecond pace. We demand the most rapid service, whether on the phone, in a restaurant, or from our family physician. We seek immediate gratification in all areas of our intensely stepped-up lives. And if we aren't getting what we want, when we want it, we become impatient, irritated, or bored.

The payoff for all that speeding up is more freedom—or so it seems. But ironically, the very liberty we seek is immediately thwarted because we don't have the time to explore it. And, unfortunately, the speed age sorely compromises the area that demands the most time: our intimate sexual relationships. Brevity of communication, heightened expectations, and shorter encounters are the hallmarks of the speed age. They are also antithetical to a healthy, intimate partnership.

While it's true that ED medication helps to overcome a physiological problem, it's the couple who must resolve their relationship issues. And that takes dedication, effort—and time.

TAKE THE TIME YOU NEED

It used to be that emotional connections were nurtured before a commitment led the way to marriage and sex. Today, to a large extent, just the opposite is true. Oftentimes, sex is at the starting gate of an encounter, with the possibility of an emotional connection growing from it. But there is an entire other world of intimacy, one that requires attention and nurturing. Doing so will provide the foundation for a stronger connection. Grounded in mutual affection and respect, it can then grow into a fully developed relationship.

Building—and maintaining—a long-lasting, satisfying partnership demands a commitment of time. But no matter how a relationship progresses, sex is a subject that a couple will have to return to over and over again. As part of the foundation of a solid bond between two people, it can function magnificently, bringing increased joy to and trust between the couple. As the sole pillar of a faltering marriage, it can be a weak link, at best. In between these two standards is an entire universe of experiences, unique to each couple.

With a new drug intervention at hand supplying the power to alter sexual compatibility, it's time to look at how men and women are reacting to this development. To a large extent, they are at a psychological crossroads in their lives.

WHAT MY PATIENTS HAD TO SAY

During the drug intervention trials, I interviewed a number of men and women, not only to gauge the physical effectiveness of the medication, but to get an idea of the psychological impact on them both.

The most immediate effect was on the men's renewed perception of themselves as fully functioning sexual beings. Story after story bore this out. One often-voiced comment was that the ED medication allowed men to bring their own personal style to their sexual encounters. With their confidence restored, they could relax and, sure that their erections wouldn't fail them, shift part of their focus to the pleasure of their partners.

One forty-one-year-old man who had injured himself in the gym and was unable to have sex for ten months told me, "I feel liberated. That's the only word for it. And because I was 'damaged' while exercising, I haven't been back to work out. I used to be so proud of how I looked; but once I was hurt I didn't care anymore. Now I feel whole again and I'm no longer fearful of the machines. I'm taking care of myself once more and I'm just so relieved that my lover didn't lose interest in me. Because of that, and the fact that I can perform again, I feel that he and I have something even better."

This man's story had a happy ending because of a supportive

partner. Sadly, that is not always the case. For many men whose erections have been lost, especially for a long period of time, suddenly being able to achieve intercourse may not be the solution to a disintegrating relationship. "It's not just a matter of having an erection and saying, 'Let's go for it, honey,' " says Robert Broad, a New York psychologist who treats many patients with sexual dysfunction issues. "First and foremost, the patient must honestly assess the general health of his sexual relationship and determine whether he and his partner are in sync and ready to work together toward the same common goals.

"Oftentimes, when the male is restored, new pressures are exerted on the relationship. Making the assumption that both partners are interested in intercourse is often a false one," says Dr. Broad. "Many men are surprised to find that their partners are not happy to resume intercourse on a regular basis. What I often hear from female patients whose husbands have been successfully treated for ED is, 'Why do I have to have sex all of the time now? I was happy the way it was.'

"There are also some women who have never viewed themselves as sexual—and prefer to stay that way. Many women are readily able to accept a partner's ED because it is more in keeping with their own sexual appetite. Some are not sympathetic to their husband's frustration at the loss of his ability—and they are not at all excited at its restoration.

"I find that the best interpersonal relationships are built upon constant communication between partners," Dr. Broad states. "Sex is not just about being good in bed or having a hard erection; rather it has to do with two people caring, caressing, and accommodating changes in the area of physical abilities. It also has to do with accepting, rejoicing in, and celebrating the all-important gender differences, recognizing, too, the uniquely different sensibilities that men and women bring to lovemaking."

People who have suffered with ED often lose sight of this, solely and unfairly equating ED with a loss of manhood. When this viewpoint is stuck in place, it is the erection—not the relationship—that becomes more important than anything else. In some cases it can irrevocably lead to an inability to trust any sexual partner, with the idea of sustaining a relationship a distant dream.

ONE MAN'S STORY

This was exactly the case with Jack, a thirty-two-year-old advertising executive whose bike accident dramatically altered his life. Riding his high-tech twenty-one-speed mountain bike in one of the many regional races he entered throughout the year, he hit a patch of gravel and started to go down. Yanking his foot from the pedal in an attempt to break his fall, he lost his balance. The next thing he was aware of was the most excruciating pain he had ever experienced—his genitals had slammed into the bike's center bar. Lying on the ground crumpled in the fetal position, he knew something bad had happened to him.

An hour later Jack saw blood in his urine and, still in agony, called his doctor, who suggested a urological examination. At the doctor's office, Jack had a complete work-up. The urologist's diagnosis was somewhat reassuring. He stated that there was no need for immediate concern, but it was still important for Jack to monitor both his urinary flow and erectile function to determine any residual damage. His urine remained clear but, two weeks later, when his fiancée came back from a business trip, he discovered the full extent of his injury, both physical and psychological.

For the eighteen months they had been together, Jack and Christina had reveled in their sexual prowess. It was a big turn-on for them both, the bond that brought and kept them together. However, on Christina's first night back something happened. Or, rather, didn't happen. For the first time in his life Jack couldn't perform. Stunned, he couldn't believe it. Neither could Christina, who, missing him for two weeks and in the mood for a prolonged sexual encounter, was both disappointed and suspicious. Becoming angry, she accused him of seeing another woman in her absence. Jack told her, as calmly as he could, what had happened to him but she didn't believe a fall could hurt him that badly.

"You've fallen off that bike before—and this never happened!" she pointed out angrily. Then, calming down somewhat, she suggested that they visit another urologist together. Unfortunately, the news they heard only contributed to the downward spiral of their relationship. The new urologist informed them that the type of bicycle accident Jack had sustained often causes mild to moderate erection difficulties, and it could take some time for full healing to take place—if it did at all. But the doctor had a recommendation: he proposed that Jack begin injecting himself with tri-mix. Then he went one step further, stating that if Jack's condition deteriorated over time, he should consider getting a penile implant.

Five months before their wedding, this news shocked them. They decided to postpone the ceremony to give them time to adjust to what would be, in both their eyes, a lifetime of artificial sex. But the adjustment never took place. Six weeks later Christina returned his ring and Jack was left alone with his problem.

Determined to prove his virility, Jack decided to use the tri-mix injections. Not wanting any woman to be aware of what he was doing, his challenge was to master the needle. Then, not satisfied with the one-hour erection the drugs gave him, he began to experiment with the dosages on his own. Figuring out a way to give himself a two-hour erection was, to him, a triumph. While demonstrating his sexual stamina fueled his badly eroded self-esteem, soothed his battered ego, and even appealed to his competitive nature, the most intimate bond he had was with his frequent injection. Ultimately, his erection—not his feelings for a woman—was the most important aspect of any sexual encounter he had.

After two years of boasting how his sexual skills were all-conquering, Jack began to feel ashamed of himself. Looking inward, he knew that he was offering women little of who he was; all that he was willing to give them was a super-hard erection. And on the flip side, what were women contributing if all their encounters were centered around how long intercourse lasted?

Realizing it was time for professional help, Jack sought out a psychotherapist who advised him to regroup, both physically and emotionally. Telling him that it would be in his best interest to cease all sexual activity for a while, the doctor said that Jack had to acknowledge the change in his erectile capabilities. In essence, he needed to take the time to mourn his loss, something he had not allowed himself to do.

Additionally, the therapist suggested that he date women with the clear understanding that sex was a boundary that was not to be crossed. This would give him time to understand that there were women who were interested in the whole person who was Jack. Over time, he began to heal and date again. He found that he was having spontaneous morning erections. When the therapist felt that he was ready, she referred Jack—and his girlfriend Gayle—to me to become part of the Vasomax trials. Interestingly, Jack wanted to first experience the effects of the medication by himself.

Observing himself respond naturally to erotic stimulation and feeling himself become hard as he masturbated was incredible to him. Then ejaculating and watching his penis retract—just as it had before the accident—made him realize two very important things. One, of course, was that for all practical purposes, he could resume a normal sex life once again. The other was that after all the emotional suffering he had endured, he now understood the value of having someone he cared about, someone with whom he could spend time and know intimately. This would make him happier than he ever thought he could be. And finally, he realized who had been missing from his sexual encounters of the past few years—himself.

With these insights, Jack was able to move forward with his psychotherapy and in his relationship with Gayle. This time, with the medication, sex was a natural outgrowth of bonding. Needless to say, it was satisfying, physically and emotionally, for both of them.

AFTER ED: A NEW BEGINNING

Jack's reaction is far from unique. In fact, I've seen men, tortured by a long history of erectile dysfunction, suddenly change after taking the medication. With the restoration of a fulfilling sex life, patients have become calmer, happier, and more optimistic about their ability to fully engage in all the aspects of their personal relationships.

One patient described it to me this way: "For the first time in three years, I was able to make love without feeling that I had to totally control the situation from start to finish. We could both relax, take our time, and enjoy being with each other. It's what sex should be."

Often, regaining erectile function gives men the confidence to enjoy other sexual activities, including prolonged foreplay, sensate touch, oral gratification, and erotic role playing. It allows them to receive pleasure more readily, and share that excitement with their partner. With the pill there is no longer any need to restrict sexual activity. Men and women can now enjoy the full repertoire of sexual expression. The magic of the medication is that it allows sex to regain its natural rhythm.

Then, too, there are those men who regard their restored function as a second chance. This time, they want to make everything as good as it can be, and share optimally with their partners on every level. To me, they express a deep sense of appreciation and gratitude—especially those who have experienced ED for long periods of time. Such patients take nothing for granted, and particularly not where their relationships are concerned. They are willing, indeed eager, to examine their feelings in ways they couldn't before because they were preoccupied with their physical states. The result, very often, is two people who are much happier. Having seen the transformative effects of the drug, the partners of these men are delighted with the changes that affect both of them.

THE FIVE KEYS TO A BETTER SEX LIFE

In order to make the most of your own "second chance," why don't you and your partner try to look inward? Bring out into the open issues that may have been lurking beneath the surface. To make your bond stronger, to create a trusting atmosphere that will foster growth, to progress to a mutually fulfilling relationship, it's time to find out how you—and your partner—feel. That covers a lot of territory, including an honest evaluation of your sex lives in five key areas that have an impact on both of you. They are:

- the meaning of sex in your relationship
- reactions to taking ED medication
- degree of personal sexual satisfaction
- identifying sexual problems
- anxieties related to intimate matters

The Meaning of Sex in Your Relationship

It is important to have a realistic understanding of the nature of your relationship with your sexual partner. A restored erection is no guarantee of improvement in a relationship that may be suffering emotionally, nor is erectile function the key to romance or monogamy. Rick's response to having ED, living with it, and finding a treatment for it provides one real-life example. At thirty-nine, he was a successful commercial photographer. Divorced, he liked a life where models posed for him during the day and succumbed to his considerable charms at night. Having a monogamous relationship was the last thing on his mind when ED brought him to my office.

"You know what it is?" he asked me, grinning slyly. "Too many women, that's what. They've just worn me out."

"How long have they been 'wearing' you down?" I wanted to know.

Looking at me sheepishly, he answered truthfully. "It's been six months."

"What happened back then?"

Thinking for a moment, Rick said, "I never considered it before, but it's when I started having insomnia. It's something I've had off and on for years, but recently it's been awful. What's really terrible is that I'm awake so much of the time—and I can't use it to have sex."

"So you were satisfied with your sex life the way it was?" I asked.

"Sure, what was not to like? I had a lot of women. I loved it—it was the way I dreamed of life being when I was a teenager."

"Then sex was the most important part of your relationship with those women?"

"What relationship? We slept together; that's what I wanted. It's what they wanted, too." Then he added, "Well, most of them. Sometimes they hinted that they wanted more; but by that time I was ready to move on anyway. But I didn't think they had anything to complain about. After all, 'satisfaction guaranteed' was my motto."

After telling Rick about the oral medications available to him he was, to say the least, ecstatic. "I can be a man again," he said. "I don't have to feel lousy anymore."

Rick's story makes it clear that, for him, sex is basically a mutually satisfying recreational activity. Consider his comments:

- he was satisfied with his sex life prior to the onset of ED and happy with his frequent partnerings
- sex was the core of his limited relationships

- he had no relationship aspirations, nor did he wish for a long-term relationship with anyone
- the thought of a renewed, invigorated sex life was all that he yearned for
- he had no inclination to change his emotional lifestyle
- he intended to continue his pre-ED sex life because it worked for him

What the medication could do was restore Rick to his pre-ED life, which was precisely what he wanted. Having been married and divorced, for the time being Rick was perfectly content with the level of intimacy he achieved during his sexual encounters. In his case, limited safe sex was the extent of the relationship he sought with a partner. Once restored, he felt that his life was again complete. "Life couldn't be better," he said. "Between the great ladies I get to meet and share some good loving with, and the wonderful family and friends that I have, what more could I want?"

There are other considerations where the meaning of sex in a relationship is concerned. Here's another case, very different from Rick's. Arthur, at fifty-seven, had been married for thirty years when his hypertension-related ED brought him and his wife, Elaine, to my office. A very handsome couple, they emanated a feeling of togetherness.

"We're really distressed at this development," Arthur began. "We've always had a good sex life and, frankly, we miss it."

Expanding on her husband's comments, Elaine added, "I have to confess—sex isn't quite as earthshaking an event for me as it is for Arthur. But I enjoy the togetherness, and I'm distressed to see him so bothered and unhappy for so long a period of time."

"Then the thought of a reinvigorated sex life doesn't bother you," I asked her.

"Oh no. In fact, I would welcome it. And if reinvigoration means what I think it does, then maybe it will do something for me, too," she answered with a blush.

Reaching over to hold her hand, Arthur told me, "I have to say that my own expectations aren't huge—but I owe it to both of us to do what I can."

This loving pair showed another dimension of a sex life:

- both partners were content with their pre-ED sex lives, but at different degrees of satisfaction
- friendship was the foundation of their relationship
- one had increased expectations, while the other did not
- they were willing to take the time to make the adjustment required
- they didn't want to keep things the way they were just because it would be simpler that way

For this couple, the pill was much more than erection insurance. They clearly saw its implications for them. They could now build on what they already had. Because their feelings and trust for each other were so strong, the medication held the promise for even greater connectedness. To them, sex was an extension of their love for each other.

Sexual expectations are not always conscious, nor are they regularly communicated to another person. As a result, partners are often at cross-purposes when their pleasure-seeking goals are on the line. That was the situation of Gina and Paul, both in their mid-thirties, who had been married for four years. Their mutual attraction had been based on their shared work—both were dedicated medical researchers—but now they seemed to be going in opposite directions.

"Ever since Paul began to experience his ED, something has

changed," Gina began. "I don't mean just the physical side; I mean the emotional one as well. He's pulled away from me. Anytime I start to talk about how I feel about our situation he walks out of the room. He's taken up a hobby—coin collecting—which he works on alone, in the middle of the night."

His face reddening, Paul replied, "That's because the last thing I want to do is discuss my erections with her. I feel strongly that it's my problem. I realize she's affected by it but I don't see how having a sensitivity session about it is going to make it any better."

"It's not going to make it worse," she pointed out.

"I disagree. The truth is—I never felt that we had such a great sex life to begin with. Now I have the opportunity to change it—"

"And you'd rather explore that brave new world with someone else," she finished the sentence for him.

As he nodded his head in assent, Gina excused herself and walked out of my office.

"I'm sorry about this," Paul told me. "It's not that I don't have feelings for Gina. It's just that we were each other's first real lover, and then we got married and spent so much time working that we—I— never had the time or inclination to explore what I really wanted from sex. I didn't even want to, until my ED occurred. Now I have another opportunity—and I want to take it."

Not surprisingly, Gina and Paul split up a short time later. The basis for their marriage—shared work—was not enough to keep them together. Sadly, their breakdown in communication prevented them from trying to find another bond to keep them together. Today, Paul's ED is under control and he is excited at the prospect of exploring his own sexuality more fully.

The emotional issues in their situation included:

• dissatisfaction of one partner with their sex lives
• a change in feelings toward a partner
• unwillingness to discuss the problem

Think about your own feelings concerning:

- how satisfied you are with your sex life
- how content you are with your present partner or partners
- how pleased your partner is with your sexual relationship
- the frequency of your sexual encounters
- what the core of your relationship is, and whether it is based on sex, friendship, or family
- your comfort level in discussing your sexual attitudes
- the reaction of your partner
- the likes and dislikes in the sexual history with your partner
- things you would like your partner to do
- things you wish your partner wouldn't do
- any changes you would like to make

Remember that a satisfying sex life is a major component of a healthy life. When the physical aspects of a relationship are on track, you and your partner are in sync. Anticipating each other's needs and wants, you create an experience that is greater than the two of you. Boosting vitality, vigor, and optimism, a mutually gratifying sex life adds to overall mental and physical contentment.

Reactions to Taking ED Medication

Some men, already on drugs to control a health problem, have no objection to taking another pill. They know that medication can help them and don't necessarily balk at having an additional prescription filled. Other men, however, have a different take on the situation. To them, their ED is terrible enough—but they believe that by toughing it out, their complete function will return. To them, medical intervention connotes "weakness"; they need the counseling of a sympathetic physician to overcome this attitude.

One man who felt that way was Thomas, a forty-eight-year-old veteran of the police department, whose stress-related ED was exacerbated by his two-pack-a-day smoking habit. Crushed by his condition, which had been present for over two years, he had been coerced by his wife to take part in the Vasomax study. Obviously uncomfortable, he crossed and uncrossed his legs as his wife began the interview. "This thing is eating him up alive," Megan began, "and it took everything I had to get him here. What he doesn't seem to realize is that I'm affected, too—as is everyone in our family. And, of course, they don't know why we argue all the time or why he's been so angry and short-tempered. Neither one of us would ever divulge something like that."

I agreed with Megan that keeping the problem between the two of them was a good idea, but that deciding to share it with a doctor was an even better one.

Thomas, however, didn't exactly feel that way. "Look—it's not personal—I have nothing against you, Doc. But I think that the job is getting to me, and after I retire in two years, everything will be the way it was. Frankly, I don't believe the drug will work." Then, turning to Megan he added, "Besides, when did you become so sex-obsessed?"

Megan rolled her eyes and addressed him. "Are you planning to stop smoking in two years, too? Your pride is getting in the way. Do you honestly think that I would feel less for you if you took medication? Face it, Thomas, you need help. We need help. Please consider trying the pills!"

He did—and was enormously relieved to regain his sexual function. However, the prior years had taken their toll and Thomas and Megan knew they had a lot of work ahead. They began to see a marriage counselor in order to salvage what they could of their damaged relationship.

The emotional issues touched upon in their case were:

- divergent views on a problem affecting them both
- a supportive partner who wanted to regain what had been lost

- acknowledgment that a restoration of sexual function wouldn't solve all their problems

Needless to say, married men, or those in committed relationships, aren't the only ones affected by ED. Single men suffer, too, and their feelings delve into another emotional arena. In Jason's case, being single complicated his ED immeasurably. A forty-three-year-old man who had never married, this landscape architect had put his dating life on hold ever since ED had become a problem. Before that, he had enjoyed the company of women. While he hadn't been searching for a commitment, he nonetheless tried to make each relationship as fulfilling as possible, both sexually and, to the extent that he was able, emotionally.

"I have to tell you," he said, "the thought of beginning a new relationship is very scary to me. I could be wrong, but I strongly feel that a woman might think less of me if I just wanted sex all the time. I like sex as much as the next guy, but I want to be more than a walking erection."

The pill worked beautifully for Jason—as soon as he found a woman he really liked and trusted.

The emotional issues in his case were:

- concern that his partner would want him just for sex
- a worry that he would, therefore, have to be in a constant state of arousal

Think about your own feelings concerning:

- erectile problems, and whether they were present at the beginning of a relationship
- the fear of losing control during sex
- whether the pill could bring you closer to your partner

- the potential sexual reaction of your partner
- the possibility that a restoration of sexual function could enhance—or threaten—your situation
- your concern about a partner's response to your sexual overtures and techniques
- how sexually demanding your partner is
- sexual desire and what it means to you
- sensory pleasure, and your capacity for it
- the difference, if any, between your anticipated relationship and how it has turned out in reality

Seriously evaluate whether you and your partner are in agreement about using the oral medications. They can affect your life in many ways and you owe it to yourselves to address issues that concern you both.

Degree of Personal Sexual Satisfaction

Any relationship is bound to have its physical ups and downs. However, a realistic appraisal of personal satisfaction is something that must be faced if a couple is to reach an enlightened connection. In the case of Rachel and Joshua, their sexual problem was, interestingly enough, related to the society in which they lived. A couple in their early twenties, they had been married for a year when they came to see me. Participants in an arranged marriage dictated by their culture, they were expected to have children as soon as possible. They told their respective families that they were seeing doctors to address their fertility problem.

Sadly, whether fertility was an obstacle was a moot question. The fact was they had only achieved intercourse a couple of times. At his young age, Joshua was experiencing erectile dysfunction.

"Our parents brought us together, we got married, and now we're expected to have children," Joshua told me with frustration rising in his voice. "We want to—of course. It's just that I can't perform regularly. I don't understand it!"

His physical exam revealed abnormally high cholesterol, which, I hastened to explain, very often contributes to ED as a man ages. I suspected that in Joshua's case, the ongoing pressure to immediately build a family might be the major culprit and I suggested a consultation with a sex therapist.

After numerous sessions, the therapist reluctantly agreed that no progress had been made. It was at this time that Joshua and Rachel enrolled in the Vasomax study.

My only concern in their case was that they had little frame of reference to compare before-and-after personal sexual experiences. "We've been together for a while now," Rachel ventured, "and, despite the problems we've been having, we've been able to get to know each other in a very positive way. What I see this pill giving us is the opportunity to build on what we've already established. If we can get over this hurdle, I'm convinced that the love and affection we have for one another will move us forward to where we want to go."

Joshua nodded in agreement. "Rachel is right. We want to get past this dark period and move on—even if it takes us a while to do it."

Happily, the pill did for them what they hoped it would, and their joint feelings made the outcome the satisfying one they were hoping for. The personal satisfaction issues in this case were:

- mutual frustration at the lack of a sex life
- shared comfort in the basic relationship, based on compatibility
- anticipation of exciting and fulfilling sexual experiences—as well as becoming first-time parents

• • •

Another view of personal gratification can be seen in the case of fifty-five-year-old Edward. Married for the third time, he was besotted with thirty-year-old Nicole, and his concern about aging motivated him to see me.

Running his hands through his steel-gray hair, Edward made his wishes known. "I'm not deluding myself. I know my personal sexual clock is ticking and it's bound to slow down. I want insurance that I can count on. The last thing in the world I want to do is disappoint Nicole and have her look to a younger man for satisfaction."

The fact that Edward was in my office alone disturbed me, and I told him so. In order to be a part of the trials, he had made an appointment for them both.

"Well, I don't want Nicole to know that I need help," Edward said. "Right now we're in a really good place, sexually, for both of us. But once in a while I'm not as hard as I'd like."

When I asked what Nicole's reaction had been on those occasions, he shrugged his shoulders. "It amazes me, but she doesn't seem to care. She had a really bad marriage when she was twenty—the guy was very abusive to her—and she says that feeling safe and loved is one of the biggest turn-ons of all, sex or no sex."

After I explained to Edward that the oral intervention could bolster his confidence as well as his erection, I made another recommendation. Given his closeness to Nicole, and her comfort with him, I strongly suggested that he speak to her first. He did, and they came in for a second visit. I prescribed the drug, and now they are prepared to override any sexual glitches that may arise in the future. The emotional issues in this case were:

- fear of incompatibility arising out of age difference
- concern about a partner's level of pleasure
- the desire for increased pleasure
- expectation of an even better relationship

Think about your own feelings concerning:

- how often you have sex and how satisfying it is for you
- restarting sexual activity where none has existed for a prolonged period of time
- whether your sexual expectations have diminished or risen
- keeping your sex-life status quo

The most fulfilling sexual satisfaction is based on an understanding of the other person's needs and desires.

Identifying Sexual Problems

This is an extremely delicate matter because it involves you and your partner at the most intimate level. Close examination of this aspect of your relationship can cause pain, no matter how gently the subject is approached. As Dr. Broad points out, "Stating your needs is critical, but be sure to choose your words carefully."

Without honesty and openness about what is making you uncomfortable or what you desire for more pleasure, you are both going to be stuck. Many times, ingrained embarrassment stemming from social or religious attitudes is the reason for silence. Most often, however, it's due to a lack of self-awareness about what makes sex personally enjoyable.

A mediator with diplomatic skills would have been a welcome addition to my meeting with Monica and Charles. Married for twenty-two years, this couple, both in their late fifties, were tense and drawn when they strode into my office.

"Let's get this charade out of the way as fast as we can," Monica began as soon as she was seated. "He wants to get his erections back—but it has nothing to do with us."

"Why should it?" Charles snapped back at her. "We've been living like brother and sister for the last six years—which predates my sex problems by four. Besides, why do you care? Sex was always a big bore to you anyway—no matter what I did to make it exciting."

In an attempt to intercede, I asked them why they were still together.

Sighing, Monica presented her side in a singsong voice that sounded as if it had been repeated many times before. "We have two children; our families would be devastated if we split up; being married is good for both of our careers. Isn't that enough?"

"Not anymore," Charles interjected. "Now there's a chance for me to have a full life again. I'm entitled to it—even if you don't think so."

Feeling his ED was in part related to his bad marriage, Charles and Monica separated. Charles took the time to discover what he really wanted, in or out of a relationship. When he did, the pills worked for him and his new partner.

This volatile situation contained several sexual problems:

- only one person wanted to make a change
- unequal interest in sex
- mutual dissatisfaction

Another instance of a couple with sexual problems was that of George and Katherine. In their early fifties, they had lived together for ten years when I saw them. George's ED, the result of surgery three years before, had put a serious damper on what had been a working relationship. However, after the pills were prescribed for him, something had changed.

"Ever since he's gotten his erections back, it's like living in a porno movie," Katherine began. "He wants to try things that make me uneasy —to say the least. And he wants to have sex a lot more frequently than we ever did before his illness. I understand—I really do—that he's overjoyed at getting back what he thought he lost forever. But still, I have to adjust to it, too, and he's not giving me the time to do it."

"Who has time?" George erupted. "We have to take what we want, when we want it. If you'd been hurt like I was, you'd *really* understand."

"Look," she told him. "I feel guilty when I tell you I don't feel like having sex. And then I feel angry when you give me grief about it."

In this situation, I referred Katherine and George to a psychotherapist. His anger and her guilt were a volatile combination, and they required professional guidance to help sort out their dilemma. In time, they were able to do so, drawing on the strong elements that had kept them together.

The sexual problems that touched them included:

- anger at a partner who refuses sex
- different ideas of appealing sexual behavior

Think about your own feelings concerning:

- any deficiency in your sex life
- your preferred sexual activities and those of your partner
- whether you perceive that you give your partner more than she gives you
- a sexual act that you would like to engage in
- any guilt felt about those acts, or ones you already perform
- your reaction when or if your partner doesn't want to have sex

Where sexual problems are present, a couple often needs outside help. If you are committed to each other, you owe yourselves the time and effort needed to pass those roadblocks in your relationship.

Anxieties Related to Sexual Matters

One of the most common obstacles to satisfying sex stems from feelings of anxiety. There are numerous causes, including fear of not being able to perform adequately, dissatisfaction with penis size, self-consciousness about body appearance (especially weight), and financial or health concerns. Sometimes fear itself is a factor.

On a strictly physiological basis, anxiety can effectively prevent a man from becoming aroused and getting or maintaining an erection. It can also limit or even destroy spontaneity and curtail the partner's exploration of new sexual territory.

Consider the case of Linda and Greg. His ED had been brought on by a combination of factors including obesity, insomnia, and stress. Sadly, all three of his conditions were a response to Linda's precarious state of health. She was diagnosed with breast cancer at the age of thirty-eight. Greg, three years older and devoted to his wife, wasn't all that surprised when his own problems began. When they came to see me two years later, their circumstances had, fortunately, changed. Linda had come through surgery and a course of radiation weak but determined. Her prognosis was excellent. Greg, however, still had his ED.

"It's not that I don't want to have erections again," he began nervously. "It's that I'm worried that after I take the medication and can function again, I'll hurt Linda. She's so thin and frail, I'm afraid to have sex with her."

"You've been scared to touch me for two years," she challenged him.

"That's because I saw what was happening to you and it put a brake on me."

Linda regarded him with a combination of sadness and anger. "I think you're just put off by how I look. Be honest, Greg—isn't it true?"

Smiling ruefully, he answered, "The truth is, I look a lot worse than you do."

Throwing her hands up in the air, Linda exclaimed, "The competition never ends. Greg, I want you to know—in front of a witness—that I want you again, spare tire and all. If you want me, then it's with my buzz cut and protruding ribs. But you have to stop being afraid of me. I'm not going to break—and you're not going to hurt me any more than I'm going to hurt you."

This situation is not an unusual one: sex is often a casualty of cancer. Please note that sex will not cause the disease to spread; nor are women who receive radiation dangerous to your health. (This is a particular concern for men whose partners have cervical cancer.)

Many patients find it difficult to speak to their physicians—and even their partners—about sex because they are so focused on surviving the disease and adhering to treatment schedules. With so much to deal with, it's not surprising that sex is low on their list of priorities.

The important thing to remember is that all humans are innately sexual, and the need for intimate expression doesn't evaporate when a disease occurs. If anything, the necessity for physical intimacy and human warmth increases. One's sexuality is an ever-present facet of the quality of life.

I'm happy to report that Greg and Linda were able to move forward with their sex lives because they had a solid foundation to build on. The anxiety issues they dealt with included:

- discomfort in sexual situations
- concern that the partner wouldn't accept physical flaws
- fear of harming the other person

Finally, there is the charming story of Jacob and Dorothy, who came to see me one day not long ago. Their story encompasses the range of sex in a relationship and merits telling. Having heard about the new medication, they wanted to see if it was right for them.

"I'm eighty-two and Dorothy is a few years younger," Jacob said. "I'll get right to the point. We have a fiftieth wedding anniversary coming up and we're booked into the bridal suite of a very grand hotel. We still remember the first time, and how wonderful it was, even though I've been less successful as of late."

"That's something we've adjusted to, but we still touch each other all the time," his wife added. "It would be wonderful if we could consummate our lovemaking more often."

"If we can have it again—even one more time to celebrate in style—we'd be so grateful," Jacob said.

Compatibility, a common sensibility, and mutual admiration are all markers of a successful partnership. As it turned out, Jacob responded extremely well to the medication, and they are still celebrating.

The emotional issues touched on here included:

- a remembered successful first sexual encounter
- a shared enthusiasm for a renewed sexual relationship
- communication, both physical and emotional

None of us is a mind reader, so I reiterate that you must communicate clearly what your sexual choices are. The first thing to do is define for yourself what satisfies you sexually. The next is to listen to what works for your partner. Adaptability and compromise are the markers of highly successful sexual relationships.

INITIATING CHANGE

It's never easy to admit that your sexual relationship needs help. Modifying it takes work and time, but knowing those areas that are giving you and your partner trouble will make it easier. Of course, each relationship is unique unto itself, as unique as the two people involved in it. But there are several general points that everyone should keep in mind:

Always Keep the Lines of Communication Open

It's paramount that you speak frankly with your partner about your condition. You must know whether each of you is supportive. Be honest about your feelings, sexual needs, and desires. If you are both in agreement that treatment is the right course, your partner needs to be part of the process.

Schedule Time for Love

Plan blocks of time, within your regular schedule, when you are both relaxed and comfortable. Recognize that as a man ages, he requires more stimulation in order to become aroused.

Work as a Team

Partners who share the goal of regaining sexual function are most likely to succeed. By working with your partner and physician, you have the best chance of regaining complete sexual fulfillment.

Consider the Benefits of Counseling

If you find that you cannot satisfactorily resolve your problems, I urge the two of you to seek additional help. Sexual counseling with a psychiatrist, psychologist, or certified sex therapist can be an effective way to strengthen and deepen a relationship while regaining lost pleasure.

I am always gratified when my patients respond positively to ED medication. But it is even more satisfying when they and their partner are able to address—and solve—any other problems in their relationships.

The New World of Sexual Medicine

STANDING ON THE threshold of an entirely different medical world—
and its implications—is no small matter for either physicians or their
patients. Apart from psychiatry, the new domain of sexual medicine is
the only other medical specialty I know of that has such a profound
impact on the whole person.

One of the most significant aspects of using the ED pill is the way
it can change a man's definition of his own sexuality. Even though the
medications affect the physical, their transformative aspects touch
upon a man's psychological and emotional makeup as well. So, simply
administering medication is just one part of the restoration process.
Understanding the underlying causes, both physical and psychological,
is another. And then there is, perhaps, the most important aspect: the
effects of the medication on a man and his partner.

Any physician practicing sexual medicine must have a clear understanding of this three-part nature of human sexual dynamics. That includes urologists, psychologists, psychiatrists, internists, and family physicians. By the manner in which they so readily bring about change, these new oral medications are forcing us to focus our attention on the more subtle areas of human sexuality, including pleasure and the nature of intimacy. How doctors and their patients handle the expectations, elations, side effects, and even fear brought about by sexual medicine is a puzzle whose pieces will be put into place far into the next century.

ED MEDICATION IS JUST THE BEGINNING

Years ago I could only hope that medical science would one day find an oral medication for erectile dysfunction. But thanks to the pioneering efforts of doctors like Adrian Zorgniotti, Ronald Virag, Gorm Wagner, Ian Osterloh, Irwin Goldstein, Harin Padma-Nathan, Tom Lue, Arnold Melman, and Raymond Rosen, sexual medicine, although still very much in its infancy, has been able to take root and flourish.

One of the most profound and far-reaching effects of the oral medications is that they are able to banish an ancient human fear. As we approach the year 2000, we can finally let go of one of man's most relentless myths. ED is no longer considered an inevitable by-product of aging. Listen to the amazed comments of one of my patients.

"I'm sixty-eight years old," Harold, a participant in my study, told me. "Gloria is fourteen years younger than I am. When we married twenty-seven years ago, I was the experienced one, and, to tell the truth, it was exciting to be the leader. But the last couple of years, all that changed. When I 'failed,' I felt that I was an old man, and a lot of my joy for living evaporated. I shut out Gloria. I knew I was doing it, and why, but I went right ahead and did it anyway. She, in turn, spent more and more time with friends. Why would she want to come home?

"But ever since I regained what I lost—and I still can't believe a pill can do that—I want to live again. And Gloria, bless her, is forgiving.

I put her through a bad time. But now it's behind us—permanently. Do you have any idea what it's like to know that you can have strong erections in your sixties or seventies or even eighties? I don't care how old I look. I feel terrific because I can do what I desire with the woman I love. Who cares about age?"

Who indeed?

SEX IN THE PEAK PERFORMANCE PERIOD

Men born between 1946 and 1964, the so-called baby boomers, are now in what I refer to as their "peak performance period," a time marked by productivity and personal fulfillment. Within my practice, many of my patients fit this profile. And while I regard the period of a man's life between the ages of thirty-five and seventy to be his best, when he is at the top of his physical, mental, and creative powers, I have seen numerous indications that this is also a time of significant erectile problems.

Now, with the advent of the erection pill, peak performers have a reliable intervention that can work for them when they need and want it. And they can use it far into their senior years. With this enormous concern lifted, these men are more confident, relaxed, and less anxious, at least sexually, about growing older. So many of these patients have expressed to me the opinion that fast lifestyles, pressured careers, and lack of down time have contributed to their ED. The pill, of course, is no cure for too intense a life—we are, after all, human and can take only so much wear and tear. But a man who feels better about himself is bound to have a positive effect on his partner, his family, his work, and the world he lives in.

But, then, having found this incredible drug, will those men want more? With expanded research, new medications are being developed, and different pathways to deliver them are being explored.

STEVEN LAMM, M.D.

THE ERECTION COCKTAIL

The question has already been raised by leading urology experts: if a man has ED, why shouldn't he take two different erection pills simultaneously, thereby producing a more potent treatment package than the one-pill regimen? In fact, the issue is not *why* two or more drugs will be prescribed to be used simultaneously by men to enhance erections, but *when* this will actually happen. It's not inconceivable that this special drug mixture, combining either Vasomax or Viagra with some newer oral medication or topical gel, will be widely used for men with moderate to severe ED.

What would happen if Viagra and Vasomax were given simultaneously? We know that each drug influences a different chemical messenger system in the body. So, in theory, once they were teamed up they could then develop greater effectiveness, possibly diminishing each other's side effects while enhancing erection capability.

Already, expert urologists are enticed by the idea because there are ample comparisons. Often, in the treatment of hypertension and certain cancers, physicians prescribe chemical "cocktails." In doing so, they combine two or more drugs in such a way that any potentially negative aspects of the stronger drugs may be offset by the positive effects of the milder ones. The end result could be an even more potent treatment that works much more effectively.

UP UNTIL NOW

The introduction of erection pills has opened the door to the pharmacological enhancement of sexual pleasure. We all know that the human reproductive system is no longer reliant solely on nature to make the decision about when, and if, pregnancy should take place. Vasectomies and birth control pills are commonplace features of our lives. New technology has stretched the years in which a woman can have a baby. Today, even post-menopausal women can have children.

By altering the procreative destinies of men and women—as they wish them to be—sex is most often about pleasure. Therefore, how can the medical establishment deny humans the right to the most exciting and fulfilling sex, including entirely restored erectile function? And, for those with "healthy" function, who is to say that it shouldn't be enhanced any further?

With the approach of rapidly evolving medical technology and newer medications, is it right to prescribe drugs for a person who isn't sick? If we look at what is demanded by healthy people, the answer is a definitive yes. We are living in an era in which the public is receptive to custom-tailored pharmacological interventions that not only fight disease but also raise and maintain the quality of their lives. Our century has been marked by the nationwide use of vaccines that prevent serious illnesses in otherwise healthy people. Standardized vaccinations and injections have rendered a number of life-threatening diseases, including measles, diphtheria, polio, tetanus, typhoid fever, and even different types of hepatitis powerless.

Medicine has responded to the clamor for rejuvenating and beautifying techniques in numerous ways. Plastic surgery, liposuction, laser resurfacing of the skin—these are just a few of the procedures available to a public that wants them. They provide a much-desired alternative to appearing older or less attractive than one wants to look. Done correctly, they don't harm—they enhance. In many cases, they help to restore confidence and make the people receiving them feel a lot better about themselves. Now, having the wherewithal to appear fit and more appealing on the outside, medical science can offer innovative methods to keep the inside running the way it should.

Currently, the Human Genome Project at the National Institutes of Health is unraveling the human genetic blueprint. In just a few years, researchers will be able to look at a man's genetic background and then choose—or even design—a drug that will correct a drooping penis or boost a waning libido.

With the dawn of the new world of sexual medicine, a more immediate question has arisen. Should a man take the pill to improve erections if he doesn't think he has ED? The issue can easily be side-stepped by saying that if a man takes the pill and his erections improve, then he had ED after all. The drug is restoring a state which would exist "naturally" if the man were free of ED. However, another way to view the issue is to ask whether the pill should be used by men with no erectile problems, as a recreational pleasure-enhancer. Who decides —the patient or the doctor?

Ultimately, they will share the decision. Making sex better denotes a hallmark in the history of modern medicine. Not so long ago, even a harmless activity like masturbation was regarded by the medical community as the first step on the road to madness. Today we can openly address sexual problems—which is the first step toward solving them. With the ED medications, we are on the next rung of the ladder. Medical science is beginning, right now, to turn erectile dysfunction into an archaic reference that will, in the near future, be as small a worry as smallpox is today.

My Own Judgment Scale

There are men who don't want to ever lose what they presently have. To that end, they are willing to do everything possible—including taking the pill. Their thinking goes like this: why shouldn't a healthy man use it to make sure he won't lose his own hard erection? This and other philosophical dilemmas raised by the pill are perplexing because they verge on areas where there are no clearly defined medical answers at this time. The oral erection drugs are so new that no one as yet has had enough experience to be able to say yes or no to their "off-label" use.

Should doctors give patients who are not suffering from ED—but who nonetheless want to maximize their peak performance in every way—access to these new medications? They have already demanded them. One of my patients, a forty-two-year-old man with no erection problems, was insistent. He stated categorically that he wanted to see if he could turn back the clock and regain the rocklike hardness he had when he was twenty. His rationale was direct. "If it's available," he said, "why shouldn't I use it, as long as it won't hurt me?"

In another significant turn of events, one of my female patients, a very attractive forty-one-year-old divorcée who had heard of the pills, wanted to know if she could get a prescription for them. "If they are all that I've heard they are, I want to keep them in the night table, next to the condoms."

A highly successful vice president of a cosmetics firm, Elizabeth was adamant about why she wanted the medication. "When I go out with a man, I'm not looking for a long-term relationship or marriage. I've already been to the altar twice; I know that being married is not right for me. However, what I do want, at the end of a pleasant evening, is good sex. Believe me, I want the man I'm with to enjoy himself, too.

"But those events are less and less frequent. From my own personal poll, I can tell you that a lot of men out there are having erectile problems. I hear a lot of excuses, from too much drink to fatigue. Those men who decide to go the distance often can't—and I'm talking a wide age range here, from thirty to sixty-five years old. I sympathize with them, I really do. But all talk and no action is frustrating. I can only imagine that it's the same for them—and probably a lot worse."

I agreed with Elizabeth that ED appears in a variety of guises. In all likelihood, the men with whom she had those disappointing inter-ludes were occasionally suffering from some degree of erectile problem but refused to admit it. Although such failures can be normal there could be an underlying ED problem. An additional factor in her case may have been Elizabeth herself, whose aggressive sexual style might have been intimidating to men experiencing even once-in-a-while failures. Performance anxiety could have been an unseen presence in those cases.

But, I informed her, the pills were only prescribed for the patient who used them. Not even a concerned wife would be able to have a prescription written in her name. More importantly, I explained that I prescribe the medication in the context of sexual medicine therapy; the pill is an integral part of a larger therapeutic process. And finally, giving a man a drug without taking a thorough medical history first is not the practice of good medicine.

THE ANXIETY FACTOR

But what about those anxiety-related situations that most men can relate to? Job performance, concern over finances, problems with teenagers at home, relationship issues with a partner—the list goes on and on, changing each day. Problems stemming from daily life are universal.

Consider the example of a thirty-four-year-old patient of mine whose job as a Wall Street trader gives him more than his share of high anxiety. It so happened that Eric's third wedding anniversary coincided with the day of a stock market freefall. That night he went home, trying to put the awful day behind him, anticipating a sexual celebration. Only, it didn't happen. There was no way that he could circumvent his worry over the events of that afternoon and the result was a disappointing evening.

When he called me the next morning, I understood why his erectile failure had occurred; so did he. Then he wanted to know if he could have a prescription for the pills for those times when he might need them. He is healthy and doesn't smoke. His drinking is limited to an occasional glass or two of wine and he exercises regularly. His ED is solely anxiety-related. Why shouldn't a man with his profile, in a loving relationship, have the fallback support he may need? Isn't his quality of life being compromised otherwise?

For Eric, and the millions of men like him who will—if they haven't already—experience anxiety-related ED, the pills can relieve worry and offer substantial piece of mind. Isn't that a valid function of medicine?

I do feel, however, that the decision to provide the medication to males who are already performing at the highest sexual levels, and who have never experienced any kind of ED, must be made on a case-by-case basis. Presently, there is a lack of scientific data to support any preventive use of the oral drug. Although controlled medical studies are being planned to measure the benefits of prophylactic use—some experts are predicting that, in the near future, the drug will be taken two or three times a week, even when a man is not engaging in sex, to ensure erectile health—we may not have definitive answers for several years.

Based on my own experiences and on the extensive reports of my fellow medical colleagues, I'm extremely pleased with the profile of the medication. With the information on hand, I can weigh the merits of the drug on a risk-to-benefit ratio on a patient-by-patient basis.

WHAT COMES NEXT?

Today, sexual medicine is a fact of life. Each of us must look both inward and outward and assess what its impact may have on our lives as one of nature's most formidable barriers falls away. As science produces more medications that were formerly not thought possible, their application will have far-reaching implications on our society. But what is so incredible at this juncture is that the ED pills conjoin sexual performance and emotions. For the first time in history, medicine has tapped into the sexual-emotional link as it pertains to sex.

Ironically, it may also be the last time.

In the upcoming years, the next generation of sexual pills will be available. They, like their groundbreaking predecessors, will allow a man to perform when he wants to, but with a very significant and potentially unsettling difference. Those pills will circumvent his "emotional system." Unlike the present oral medications which require a physical attraction to a partner, those newer drugs may not. Some may affect chemicals in the brain, as opposed to the present pills which work in the penis. Other experimentation is ongoing. Studies currently being conducted may provide gene therapy to control ED via injections administered two or three times a year.

All of these interventions bring us to a new place in our culture. Today, we are on the cusp of a sexual revolution whose implications we can only begin to imagine. Those effects, both long- and short-range, are going to have a mighty impact on both sexes. Men have their own problems and perspectives about ED and its treatment. For women, however, there are different considerations and worries.

We know that the lives of millions of women have been altered by ED. So, it is very important to acknowledge that its presence and treatment can touch a woman in profound, and even disturbing, ways. For many women, this is the second time they have to deal with a pill that affects their own sexuality. Only this time, a man is taking it.

WOMEN AND THE "OTHER" PILL

When birth control pills became widely available, they sent a ripple effect throughout our society. For the first time, women could not only reliably avoid the risk of pregnancy, they had, in essence, the freedom that men had to have sex whenever they wanted it. The miracle they had dreamed about didn't cause a disruption the way other methods of birth control did. And the pill was easy to use. All a woman had to do was remember to take it.

For others, however, it had different implications. Its use brought up questions about vulnerability, self-esteem, and attractiveness. Sex before any notion of commitment was made possible by the pills. With the license to have "safe" intercourse (a very different term twenty years ago, meaning without the risk of pregnancy), a woman could enjoy, at least in theory, uncomplicated sex. But, as we know, sex is never an uncomplicated matter.

I'm drawing a comparison between birth control pills and the oral intervention for ED for very specific reasons. Ironically, the problems that now afflict men with ED may soon have an unprecedented impact on their partners. Those very questions that haunt men concerning confidence, sex appeal, and worthiness could easily be transferred to women once the pill is a part of their lives. The inevitable question will arise: "Is it the pill that's turning him on—or is it me?"

Consider the comments from Leslie, a thirty-eight-year-old woman whose ten-year marriage was at a crossroads. "Will says he's overjoyed that he can get the kind of erections he used to have. But we've been through too many tough times; we've fought a lot. He complained about the weight I gained, not realizing that it was in response to his not wanting to have sex with me. Of course, for a very long time I didn't know—because he didn't tell me—that he *couldn't* have sex. I felt so rejected, food was my only consolation.

"Now he wants to have sex again. I have to ask myself: does he still care for me, or is it just that he hasn't been able to have sex for a long time, wants to play catch-up, and is worried about straying from home and contracting AIDS? He's so enraptured with his erections, I can't honestly believe that they have much—if anything—to do with me. It makes me feel angry and used, and less attractive than ever."

Leslie's view is understandable, especially in the context of the way women judge themselves in our culture. Sadly, many women, beginning early in their lives, regulate their self-esteem through how they see their bodies, or think other people judge their physical attractiveness. We see evidence of this everywhere. Losing weight is a national obsession, supermodels are ideals for young girls, and prepubescent female athletes, many whose growth and menstrual cycles are stunted, are heroes for impressionable children.

Aging is, for many women, an enemy that must be fought at all costs. Looking and feeling the best they can while accepting their age is not their goal. Instead, beating the clock is, no matter how much self-esteem is sacrificed in the process. When self-value is solely reliant on the reactions of others to how one looks, problems are inevitable. Certainly ours isn't the first culture to put such emphasis on looks. However, the advent of a new world of sexual medicine is bound to exert more pressure on the way women view their appeal, both physically and emotionally.

According to psychologist Dr. Robert Broad, at New York's Mount Sinai Hospital, "In our society, how a woman attracts and arouses a man is a primary source of self-esteem. That initial appeal is often based on how a woman looks. This component of self-evaluation is a key factor to how a woman will respond to a man with erectile dysfunction—and how she will feel about herself."

The more vulnerable a woman feels—regardless of her age—the more she will question herself, both as the source of a man's ED and as the object of his attention.

THE WOMEN'S RESPONSE

For women without a steady partner, the occurrence of ED can be startling and unexpected, to say the least. Few women are prepared to deal with it since it is the rare man who will tell a date beforehand that he has erectile problems, whether they happened only once or are a part of his daily life. One of my female patients put it this way. "I'm twenty-five years old," Sandy told me. "I work out at the gym three times a week so I'll stay in shape. I'm really aware of how I look, and I like it when men are attracted to me. But then I went out with Sam a few times and he couldn't get it up. I couldn't believe it—he's only two years older than I am! It's just impossible for me to believe that a guy that young could have erection problems. It made me angry, and then I found myself not liking him as much as I thought I did."

Sandy's reaction was based on her own narcissism; she fully expected a peer to have as much control over his own body as she did hers. When I informed her about the new oral medications for ED, she was skeptical. "I don't see how that can change anything for us," she stated emphatically. "He needs help, but I'm not going to be the one to tell him where to get it. I'm sorry to sound so unsympathetic about it, but now he's not so appealing to me. It's like all those muscles he's been building are fake."

Then there is the perspective of Angela, a thirty-three-year-old whose six-month relationship with Pete was marked by his ED right from the start. "I know it might sound odd," she told me, "but Pete's condition didn't bother me that much; in fact, it drew me to him. I felt sorry for him and I was happy to be sympathetic. And despite his problem, he did everything he could to satisfy me sexually. I mean, it was a good situation for me—and he certainly didn't seem to mind. But now that this pill is available I'm uncomfortable. I don't want to change what we have."

In this case, Angela's narcissism is fed through her role of caretaker. It's not surprising that she feels threatened by something that can supplant that role and remove her position as sexual superior.

Single women, whether they are just beginning a new relationship or have been seeing a man for a while, should be aware of the new medications. While it's probable that ED has not yet touched their lives, it's just as likely that, at some point, it will. But at the same time, they need to take a look inside and ask themselves what they really want from a relationship.

For women in long-term relationships, ED brings numerous problems, as well as opportunities. As Dr. Broad points out, "If physical attractiveness and sexuality have been the main glue of the relationship, then the narcissistically vulnerable woman may instantly doubt her worth as a human being. Fear of abandonment, staved off while the relationship was predictable and viable, may suddenly surface when the partner develops ED."

This perspective was voiced by Amanda, a forty-eight-year-old woman who worried that her husband, Jeff, would blame his ED on her and leave. "He'll find a younger woman, I know he will," she told me. "We were such a great-looking couple—everybody said so. But now, after three children and twenty years of marriage I look different. He won't respond to me anymore. I know he's halfway out the door."

Another outlook was stated by Joan, a very wealthy woman whose marriage to Victor was one of convenience. "I know he had a girlfriend before his ED kicked in. Frankly, it never bothered me. Sex isn't a big part of our marriage. I expect him to accompany me when I need him —but then he's on his own. Now he wants to spend all his time with me, which isn't a part of our deal. We have what I think of as a business arrangement—not an emotional one."

Both these women are intent on focusing solely on their own perspectives. Because they won't—or can't—consider the causes of their husbands' ED, much less the emotional underpinnings of their marriages, they're unable to figure out what to do. As Dr. Broad states, "For these women, ED is not a sign that their partners—or their relationship—is in crisis. Rather, they experience the ED as an injury to their self-esteem. The major failure of their partners is that they can't function in a way that enhances their own self-esteem."

What happens, then, when a solution to ED is readily at hand?

WHEN THE PILL IS A THREAT

For women who are drawn to men they feel they can rescue, the pill can be perceived as a danger to the relationship. These women believe that the men's problem is the cement that keeps them together. In their private estimation, their men are "flawed," and therefore worthy of deep pity and a lot of forbearance. What this serves is the women's ego, since it makes them feel as if they are caretakers in the situation. More significantly, it also reassures them, making them secure in the belief that no man with ED will ever abandon them. After all, they rationalize, who else would want those "damaged" goods?

With their ingrained habits, women like these are generally unreceptive to their partners receiving successful treatment. They may suggest that the pills aren't safe, or that they haven't been proven absolutely effective. Under the guise of caring, they might undermine what could very well be the salvation of a partner's life in order to ensure their own perceived sanctuary. In their eyes, a restored partner is a danger to the status quo. Conceivably, they could lose their power base, their status as saint, and, ultimately, be left alone permanently.

Sadly, they are short-changing themselves. Without looking at the dynamic between the two of them, including fears, hopes, and everything in between, there is little chance that their relationships can be salvaged—much less grow to their full potential.

SYMPTOM CHECKLIST

Anger, disappointment, sadness, concern, and the urge to help are all appropriate reactions to ED. These feelings apply whether a woman is encountering a male with ED for the first time or whether the condition is within the context of an ongoing relationship. However, when living with his disorder begins to produce disruptive physical and emotional symptoms in her, it's time for a woman to seek professional help.

A symptom checklist follows. Some of these symptoms may have causes other than your partner's ED, but are nevertheless having a negative impact on your relationship.

The symptoms are:

❑ Anger	❑ Troubling thoughts
❑ Sleep problems	❑ Depression
❑ Fearfulness	❑ Anxiety
❑ Eating problems	❑ Alcohol or drug use
❑ Stress	❑ Problems at work
❑ Difficulty concentrating	❑ Memory loss
❑ Lack of self-esteem	❑ Distractedness
❑ Feelings of hopelessness	❑ Health problems

If a woman identifies more than three of the above symptoms in her partner, she should consider seeking professional help. Having a relationship with a man suffering from ED is no easy matter. Talking over the problem, and how it makes her feel, is a big step toward helping herself, as well as her partner.

WHEN THE PILL IS SALVATION

If couples cannot talk to each other about the effects that ED is having on their relationships and their lives, they should seek psychological help. At the other end of the relationship spectrum are the majority of people I see. For them, the availability of the pill has prompted the most heartfelt and honest self-evaluations I have ever heard.

One of the most memorable examples of this was articulated by Janice, a forty-five-year-old woman who was about to be married for the first time when her fiancé, Vincent, began to experience ED. They came to my office and Janice offered a keen insight into what kind of person she was and the bond she and Vincent shared.

"Vincent says that we should delay our marriage, that he's having second thoughts and doesn't want me to be saddled with a man who is 'defective,' " she said. "I'm trying to make him understand that, to me, he's a hell of a lot more than just stud service. We've been together for two years. During that time we've traveled, met each other's friends and family, and discovered what we like—and dislike—about each other. Then, last year, my mother became very ill. It was a very rough time for me and my family, and Vincent was there, every step of the way. And when she died, he gave me the kind of support I hope everybody gets at a time like that. I'll never forget it, and I'll never leave him when he needs my help."

For Janice and Vincent, whose bond is based on growing together, the pill offers another opportunity to build on an already solid foundation. Because their self-esteem is not moderated by selfish motives, they can share the problem and revel in its solution. They are now happily married. The pills prescribed for Vincent have made a satisfying relationship that much better.

But what do you do if your partner won't see a doctor?

THE IMMOVABLE OBJECT

It's no secret that men don't visit doctors as often as women. My female patients are up front about their belief in yearly checkups or, as some refer to it, "general maintenance." If you are a woman whose partner has ED and you want to help him, there are ways to do it. But in order to avoid conflict, the first thing you need to do is be sympathetic—

without anger. Point out that your overriding concern is his health, and that your love for him is making you speak. That should get his attention.

Take the time to make a list of the things he does—or doesn't do —that could potentially be harming his health. Talk to him about these issues, calmly and rationally. Discussing one or two at a time will make it more manageable. Remind him that ED is often a symptom of a physical problem or underlying medical condition that might need to be treated.

Anticipate his denials, as well as his defense mechanisms. It's unlikely that he will agree with you, especially at first. He might very well feel overwhelmed, worried, and upset that you are crossing his personal boundary. But persevere. His health, as well as your relationship, is at stake. And, of course, once he is willing to discuss his problem, your *shared* problem, then it is time to bring up the fact that he can be helped. But do keep in mind that one conversation is not likely to get him to pick up the phone and make a doctor's appointment. Both of you have to want help. And for the pills to function optimally, both of you have to want them to work—physically and emotionally.

Counteracting the ED Effects of Prescription and Over-the-Counter Medications

NOW THAT WE know that ED can be triggered by physical and psychological factors, it's time to address its very prevalent third cause, one that is, perhaps, the most insidious of all. Ironically, ED can also be brought on by what are called iatrogenic causes. This is the erectile dysfunction that is directly induced or exacerbated by physician-prescribed drugs. To that long list, we also have to add over-the-counter medications.

THE PRESCRIPTION DRUG EFFECT

Every drug has its own profile of strengths and weaknesses. While a pill may be hailed as the miracle cure of the moment, the substance will, inevitably, house a less than desirable downside. Because of this, physicians must weigh the risk-to-benefit ratio before they prescribe any medication.

Each year, doctors in this country write more than 1.5 billion prescriptions—about six per person. Although many men are simply not aware of the fact—and this often includes their physicians as well —scores of the most commonly prescribed drugs have been implicated, or at least strongly suspected, in either the development or worsening of ED. In fact, of the ten most widely prescribed drugs in use in the United States today, I have seen eight either produce or increase ED. A list of these most widely prescribed drugs was published in the November 23, 1997, issue of *The New York Times*; they are: Prilosec, Prozac, Zantac, Zocor, Epogen, Zoloft, Paxil, Norvasc, Vasotec, and Procardia. Only Epogen and Prilosec are not known to inhibit sexual function.

There is a simple explanation why a prescription drug taken to control an allergy, depression, or hypertension gives a man erectile problems. Those medications, which affect the vascular system, including blood pressure, the heart, and the respiratory organs, will have an impact on any blood-delivering system in the body. Some hamper the blood vessels in the penis by constricting them, thereby making it virtually impossible to achieve an erection. Others affect the nerves which activate penile responsiveness. Then there are the medications which strike the areas of the brain where desire and sexual pleasure are centered, resulting in a severe decrease in sex drive.

But even if you are taking a medication that you think may be causing your ED, it's imperative that you consider other possible contributing factors as well. Many times ED turns out to be the manifestation of a complex interaction among several elements, all of which need to be examined. They include:

- what the drug is for, and what dosage is being taken
- your psychological state
- the status of your relationship with a partner

It's also very important to remember that every drug affects the person taking it differently. Taking a medication at one point in a man's life may not induce ED, while it might very well at another juncture. That's why it's crucial that you personally consider, and talk to your doctor about, all the contributing factors listed above. Also, you must give the drug a chance to work and see if its side effects are temporary or not. As a rule of thumb, I recommend using the medication for several weeks before assessing its role in any ED that might develop.

THE PRIMARY OFFENDERS

If you need drugs for cardiovascular disease, diabetes, or high blood pressure, your susceptibility for erectile dysfunction is greater than in the general population. The medications which are frequently prescribed for these conditions unfortunately also contribute to the problem.

Research supports this. The Massachusetts Male Aging Study (MMAS) conducted in 1994 found that men taking vasodilator medication for their heart conditions were four times as likely to have moderate or complete ED compared to other men. Those who took cardiac drugs as well as those who needed drugs to control their diabetes were three times as likely to suffer from significant ED. And in addition, those who required medication for hypertension suffered significantly from erection problems. Cholesterol-lowering drugs are also the culprits where sexual function is concerned. While this was not apparent in the men sampled in the MMAS, I see it too often in my own practice to discount it.

Overall, there are five main classes of drugs responsible for negative sexual side effects. They are:

- *Cardiovascular drugs* for heart disease, hypertension, and elevated cholesterol.
- *Psychiatric medications,* including antidepressants, antianxiety drugs, and tranquilizers.
- *Antihistamines,* including drugs for allergies and motion sickness, and cold remedies.
- *Gastrointestinal medications* formulated to relieve heartburn, stomach aches and pain, spastic colon and bowels, and flatulence.
- *Miscellaneous drugs* which encompass substances used to treat everything from muscle spasm and Parkinson's disease to glaucoma and prostate tumors.

Let's look at each category—it's likely that you'll recognize more than a few drugs on the following lists.

Cardiovascular Medications

When hypertension is present, blood pressure stays elevated all the time at 140 millimeters of mercury (mm Hg) over 90 mm Hg or higher, putting extra pressure on the heart and arteries. In turn, the pressure can damage the surface of blood vessels and may lead to cholesterol deposition, thereby further narrowing pathways and blocking blood flow to the spongy tissue of the penis. And if a man has a high cholesterol count, the risk of penile blockage is increased because plaque will form where an artery has been damaged by high blood pressure.

Almost every antihypertensive medication is linked to some form of sexual disorder, but some are more likely than others to cause specific problems. I often use diuretics, such as chlorthalidone and hydro-chlorothiazide, as a first line of attack to lower blood pressure. In my practice, three quarters of the men taking these medications do not experience ED. However, for the quarter who do, I may prescribe an ACE (angiotensin-converting enzyme) inhibitor, such as Accupril or Vasotec, or possibly a calcium channel blocker, such as Norvasc or Procardia XL. I would tend to shy away from medications such as clonidine (Catapres), methyldopa (Aldomet), or reserpine (Hydropres). These drugs are known to have more significant ED effects.

Beta-blocker medications, which include atenolol (Tenormin), bi-soprolol (Ziac), metoprolol (Lopressor), nadolol (Corgard), propranolol (Inderal), and timolol (Blocadren) reduce the workload on the heart and, therefore, the arteries. I commonly prescribe these drugs for the treatment of a variety of cardiac problems, from coronary artery disease to hypertension. However, I've found that patients often complain of ED after using these drugs. If that's the case, I'll switch them to either a calcium channel blocker or an ACE inhibitor.

If a man has already developed ED due to an underlying medical condition, such as diabetes, or had instances of ED because of a diuretic medication he may have taken, then I will not recommend a beta-blocking drug as a first-line treatment or even as an alternative. Again, it's the ACE medication or calcium channel blocker that I would pre-scribe. ACE inhibitors are one of the most commonly used classes of antihypertensives although, to date, no one is quite sure exactly how they work. It is suspected that they block an enzyme that is required for blood vessels to constrict. As a result, the vessels relax, which is favorable to erectile function. Of the heart medications, the ACE inhibitors—benazepril (Lotensin), captopril (Capoten), enalapril (Vasotec), fosinopril (Monopril), lisinopril (Zestril), quinapril (Accupril), and ramipril (Altace)—are least likely to create ED problems.

The following chart lists the various cardiovascular medications linked to ED.

Brand Name	Generic Name
Aldactazide	Hydrochlorothiazide
Aldactazide	Spironolactone
Aldactone	Spironolactone
Aldoclor	Methyldopa
Aldomet	Methyldopa
Aldoril	Methyldopa
Atromid-S	Clofibrate
Apresazide	Hydrochlorothiazide
Blocadren	Timolol maleate
Catapres	Clonidine hydrochloride
Combipres	Clonidine hydrochloride
Crystodigin	Digitalis
Demi-Regroton	Chlorthalidone
Dibenzyline	Phenoxybenzamine hydrochloride
Diupres	Reserpine
Diuril	Chlorothiazide
Dyazide	Hydrochlorothiazide
Esidrix	Hydrochlorothiazide
Esimil	Guanethidine sulfate
Harmonyl	Rauwolfia serpentina
HydroDIURIL	Hydrochlorothiazide
Hydropres	Hydrochlorothiazide
Hygroton	Chlorthalidone
Inderal	Propranolol
Inderide	Propranolol
Ismelin	Guanethidine sulfate
Lanoxicaps	Digoxin
Lanoxin	Digoxin
Lopressor	Metoprolol
Metatensin	Reserpine
Moduretic	Hydrochlorothiazide
Norpace	Disopyramide phosphate
Oretic	Chlorthalidone

Brand Name	Generic Name
Raudixin	Rauwolfia serpentina
Rauzide	Rauwolfia serpentina
Regroton	Reserpine
Salutensin	Reserpine
Ser-Ap-Es	Hydrochlorothiazide
Serpasil	Reserpine

Psychiatric Medications

ED is not only one of the most troubling side effects of many psychiatric drugs, it is also the least discussed. "I thought it was just me," a patient said after learning that an antidepressant that he had been taking daily for two years caused his ED. "I was embarrassed to talk to you about it. And I didn't know if there was anything you could do for it, anyway."

If ED is going to become a problem for men undergoing pharmacotherapy with tranquilizers or antidepressants, the trouble usually begins during the first month of treatment. For many men who experience this initial side effect, and then stay on the program long enough to benefit from diminished anxiety and/or reduced depression, there will eventually be a reawakening of sexual interest and, consequently, improved sexual performance.

Over time, however, the sexual picture may change, again because of the drugs. Many of the treatments for psychiatric-related disorders negatively affect sexual response by impacting the autonomic nervous system, which controls the genitals. Other psychiatric drugs can block nerve function, making it difficult, or even impossible, to achieve an erection or ejaculation. High doses of tranquilizers prescribed for anxiety and depression not only cause ED, they can also be responsible for the lessening of libido (sexual desire), an inability to ejaculate, and gynecomastia (breast enlargement in men).

The popular new class of depression-fighting drugs, SSRIs, such as fluoxetine and sertraline, also inhibit sexual function. SSRIs are selective serotonin-reuptake inhibitors, a group of drugs which affect the neurotransmitter, or brain chemical, serotonin, which affects mood. These medicines often contribute to ED, diminish sex drive, and block orgasm. This latter problem is so widespread with Prozac, Paxil, and Zoloft, three of the most widely used SSRIs, that I often prescribe low dosages of them to men complaining of premature ejaculation. Current estimates of men taking SSRIs who have erectile problems range from 9 percent to 24 percent.

While it sometimes happens that sexual problems diminish after a man has adjusted to the drug he is taking, it is usually the exception to the rule. Taking a drug "holiday," or having sex when the drug is at its lowest concentration in the body, are alternatives that work for some men (see pages 165 and 166–68). For others, yohimbe (the pulverized bark of an African tree, available in health food stores or by prescription) or red ginseng can alleviate ED when taken in combination with their SSRI medications. Many of my patients have responded very well to changing from Prozac to either Wellbutrin or Serzone.

The following chart lists the various psychiatric medications linked to ED.

Brand Name	Generic Name
Anafranil	Clomipramine hydrochloride
Aventyl	Nortriptyline
Compazine	Prochlorperazine
Deprol	Meprobamate
Elavil	Amitriptyline
Endep	Amitriptyline
Equagesic	Meprobamate
Equanil	Meprobamate
Eskalith	Lithium carbonate
Etrafon	Amitriptyline
Haldol	Haloperidol

Brand Name	Generic Name
Inapsine	Droperidol
Innovar	Droperidol
Janimine	Imipramine
Librium	Chlordiazepoxide
Limbitrol	Amitriptyline
Lithane	Lithium carbonate
Lithobid	Lithium carbonate
Lithonate	Lithium carbonate
Lithotabs	Lithium carbonate
Ludiomil	Maprotiline hydrochloride
Marplan	Isocarboxazid
Matulane	Procarbazine hydrochloride
Mellaril	Thioridazine
Meprospan	Meprobamate
Miltown	Meprobamate
Nardil	Phenelzine sulfate
Navane	Thiothixene
Norpramin	Desipramine
Pamelor	Nortriptyline
Parnate	Tranylcypromine sulfate
Paxil	Paroxetine
Permitil	Fluphenazine
Pertofrane	Desipramine
Prolixin	Fluphenazine
Prozac	Fluoxetine
Serax	Oxazepam
Serentil	Mesoridazine
Sparine	Promazine
Stelazine	Trifluoperazine
Surmontil	Trimipramine maleate
Taractan	Chlorprothixene
Thorazine	Chlorpromazine
Tofranil	Imipramine

Brand Name	Generic Name
Tranxene	Clorazepate dipotassium
Triavil	Amitriptyline
Valium	Diazepam
Valrelease	Diazepam
Vivactil	Protriptyline hydrochloride
Zoloft	Sertraline

Antihistamine Medications

Developed more than fifty years ago to block the release of histamines from cells, these drugs are widely available in both prescription and over-the-counter forms. They work by counteracting the body's reaction to allergens, the ordinarily harmless substances which trigger the immune system to produce antibodies to destroy them. When you're prone to allergies, a special type of antibody, called IgE, is produced, making you super-sensitive to the allergen. Each time you're exposed to the offending substance, it combines with the IgE antibodies, releasing histamines that bring on sneezing, watery eyes, and runny noses.

Antihistamines, which dry mucous membranes, can also be responsible for ED as well as a drop in libido. I have had success with patients who switched from antihistamines to Nasalcrom or Flonase nasal spray. These medicines control allergic symptoms without affecting sexual function.

The following are drugs with antihistamine activity (allergy remedies, cold drugs, motion sickness pills, and sleeping aids) that may cause ED.

Brand Name	Generic Name
Ambenyl	Diphenhydramine
Antivert	Meclizine

Brand Name	Generic Name
Benadryl	Diphenhydramine
Benylin	Diphenhydramine
Bonine	Meclizine
Bromanyl	Diphenhydramine
Dramamine	Dimenhydrinate
Dytuss	Diphenhydramine
Mepergan	Promethazine
Nico-Vert	Dimenhydrinate
Phenergan	Promethazine
Synalgos	Promethazine
Vistaril	Hydroxizine

Gastrointestinal Medications

In a recent national survey of some of the sixty million Americans who complain of heartburn at least once a month over one third responded that the condition interfered with their sex lives. The culprit could very well be the over-the-counter medications they take for their painful symptoms.

Most antacids, such as Alka-Seltzer and Tums, contain a buffer that helps to quell stomach acid. They offer relief and don't affect erection capability. However, the newer antacids, such as Tagamet HB, Pepcid AC, Axid AR, and Zantac 75—each a former prescription ulcer medication—can. They effectively short-circuit histamine signals that are sent out after an offending food is eaten. No stomach acid means no heartburn, gas, or belching. Unfortunately, while they block stomach acid these drugs also effectively hinder the effects of testosterone, leading to a lessening of libido as well as erection difficulties.

The following is a listing of some of the gastrointestinal drugs that may cause ED problems.

Brand Name	Generic Name
Antrocol	Atropine
Arco-Lase	Atropine
Axid AR	Nizatidine
Pepcid AC	Famotidine
Pro-Banthine	Propantheline bromide
Reglan	Metoclopramide
Tagamet HB	Cimetidine
Zantac 75	Ranitidine hydrochloride

Miscellaneous Medications

The following is a list of other widely used drugs that can bring on or affect ED.

Brand Name	Generic Name	Prescribed For
Accutane	Isotretinoin	Acne
Akineton	Biperidin	Parkinson's disease
Amicar	Aminocaproic acid	Bleeding
Antabuse	Disulfiram	Alcoholism
Artane	Trihexyphenidyl	Parkinson's disease
Cogentin	Benztropine	Parkinson's disease
Diamox	Acetazolamide	Glaucoma
Dilantin	Phenytoin	Seizure
Estrace	Estradiol	Prostate disease
Eulexin	Flutamide	Prostate disease
Fastin	Phentermine hydrochloride	Appetite suppressant
Flagyl	Metronidazole	Fungal infection
Flexeril	Cyclobenzaprine	Muscle spasm
Indocin	Indomethacin	Arthritis
Kemadrin	Procyclidine	Parkinson's disease
Lopid	Gemfibrozil	Lipid lowering
Lupron	Leuprolide	Prostate disease
Norflex	Orphenadrine	Muscle spasm

Brand Name	Generic Name	Prescribed For
Norgesic	Orphenadrine	Muscle spasm
Proscar	Finasteride	Prostate disease
Sansert	Methysergide	Headaches
Satric	Metronidazole	Infection
Timolol	Beta-adrenergic blocking agent	Glaucoma
Zoladex	Goserelin	Prostate disease

YOUR PERSONAL DRUG ASSESSMENT

If you're wondering what medicines to avoid, there is no simple answer. Many drugs can affect the capacity for erections and sexual response. But if you are suddenly experiencing sexual problems, you can do some detective work on your own. And one of the first places to look is inside the medicine cabinet. Don't overlook drugs that are supposed to treat body parts unrelated to sexual function.

It was painful heartburn and the overdosing of Tagamet that brought George to my office. Wanting instant relief from his discomfort, and finding no help with the recommended dosage, the fifty-two-year-old man doubled the number of tablets. And although he felt better, he was now experiencing another problem. Suddenly, he could no longer sustain an erection. He thought he was going through "andropause," the so-called male menopause.

It didn't take long to determine what was causing George's ED. It was the massive dosages of Tagamet. However, we also needed to find out what was giving him such intense gastric problems. A simple blood test revealed the presence of an alarmingly high amount of *Helicobacter pylori* (*H. pylori*) bacteria. Typically acquired in childhood, *H. pylori* has been implicated in ulcers, cancer of the stomach and upper intestine, as well as a host of gastrointestinal ailments. George's stomach distress was being caused by a previously undiagnosed and therefore untreated peptic ulcer—not heartburn. While the Tagamet helped to reduce some of the harsher and more uncomfortable symptoms of his ulcer, it also gave him ED.

I switched George to Prilosec, a powerful acid reducer not known to be associated with ED in combination with an effective antibiotic to knock out the *H. pylori*. After thirty days, George was symptom- and medication-free. His ulcer, as well as his erection problem, were gone.

USING YOUR ED DRUG CHART

Keep in mind that you must give a new drug a few weeks to work before you can determine if it is causing your problems. If you have begun a new course of medication and suspect that it might be giving you ED, continue with it—but be sure to discuss your concerns with your doctor. If the lines of communication between you and your doctor are kept open, it is usually possible to change or adjust medication. The goal is to maintain your general health while not adversely affecting your sexual performance.

The chart presented here is designed to help you pinpoint whether a specific drug you're taking is causing ED. It includes:

Name of the Medication

Under this heading, list every drug you are taking by brand and generic name. Include any over-the-counter drug as well.

The Prescribing Physician, Diagnosis, and Date Medication Was Started

This becomes especially important as you develop more ailments and consult with different doctors.

Dose and Frequency

In order for a drug to work effectively, you have to know the correct dosage, how often it should be taken, and when.

Adverse Side Effects

Have your doctor or pharmacist explain the major side effects of the drug to determine if ED is a possible outcome.

Sexual Difficulties

If you develop ED, or if it has worsened since beginning the medication, note it on your chart. Include any performance problems like lessened libido or delayed orgasm. Your symptoms may be related to the new drug. Ask your doctor if a different drug can be substituted, or if a lower dose could be used to eliminate, or at least reduce, the sexual dysfunction.

Drug Efficacy

This is the place to write down if you feel the drug is working and fully achieving the projected goal.

The following chart is that of a patient who received a new drug to help reduce his hypertension. As you will see, it didn't work for him. After a month, his medication was changed, the side effects were significantly reduced, and his sexual problems disappeared.

Name of medication (generic and brand names)	Doctor, diagnosis, date started	Dose and frequency	Adverse side effects	Sexual difficulties	Drug efficacy
Diuretic Chlorthalidone	Lamm, hypertension: 175/105, 6/3/97	50 mg once a day	electrolyte imbalance, fever, chills, low back pain, possible ED	erection problem: 6/19/97 6/30/97	No

Note: Keep track of how much alcohol and/or tobacco you use on a daily basis as they too can contribute to, or produce, ED.

THE MEDICAL OPTIONS: AVOIDING ED AS A SIDE EFFECT

It is a challenge to effectively treat a health-compromising ailment while at the same time circumventing ED. However, there are ways that it can be done. I have implemented all of the following six options, where appropriate:

1. Changing the medication to one that has the same capabilities but is less likely to trigger ED.
2. Lowering the dosage of the medication and observing whether the health condition is still controlled and ED either diminishes or disappears.
3. Decreasing the medication's dosage and adding another low-dose drug to help control the underlying primary medical condition.
4. Taking a drug "holiday," if suitable to the case.
5. Constantly being alert to newer treatment options.
6. Timing a patient's sexual activity to the medication's lowest strength during a twenty-four-hour period.

To illustrate these methods, here are examples of how each one worked for six different patients.

Option 1: Changing Medications

Harold, at fifty-five, had a dangerously high cholesterol count of 300 milliliters, coupled with a very low HDL of 25 milligrams. (It's important to note that both high cholesterol and low HDL are markers of ED.) I began him on a course of Mevacor, a cholesterol-lowering agent, and his reading soon dropped to 220. Unfortunately, he also developed ED. Understandably upset, Harold wanted to try other medications.

At his next visit I recommended that he switch to prescription niacin (which is not found in health food stores). While this proved to be an effective treatment for both his cholesterol and erection problems, there were other unpleasant side effects to confront: abnormal liver function and facial flushing. Fortunately, there was another alternative. Harold began to take Cholestid, a bile-acid resin, and in a couple of months his cholesterol stabilized at 210, and his HDL levels rose to a much-improved 41. His liver function was normalized, and the new cholesterol-lowering drug did not produce any erection problems.

Option 2: Lowering the Dosage

Roger, at forty-nine, was a twenty-eight-year veteran of the New York police force. Years of desk work had contributed to poor circulation, varicose veins, and chronic edema of the legs. When he first came to see me, he complained of leg swelling and intolerable itching. To relieve his symptoms, I prescribed 40 mg of Lasix, an often-used diuretic, and suggested that he begin a regular walking program to improve circulation. I also recommended that he cut back substantially on the processed meat sandwiches he often ate—they are infamous water retainers. He also took regularly scheduled breaks from his desk for badly needed stretches and new leg positions.

When I saw him five months later, his condition had greatly improved, but now he had a new complaint: periodic episodes of ED. Since he had responded so well to Lasix and had incorporated lifestyle changes into his daily routine, I decided to try lowering his dosage. The intention, of course, was to maintain his improved circulation as well as combat his ED. First, he tried taking the medicine every other day instead of daily. The result was a return of the edema and sporadic

ED. The next step was to reintroduce the daily dose, but at lower levels. This time, the edema was reduced and the ED was eliminated.

Option 3: Lowering the Dosage and Adding Another Drug

Bill was taking 100 mg of Hygroton, a diuretic used to lower his hypertension. Although the medicine worked, the forty-six-year-old soon developed erection problems. To counteract his ED, I chose to lower the dosage to 25 mg, although I knew that this alone would not be enough to control his blood pressure. So, I also prescribed a small dose of Hytrin, a vasodilator. The combination of the two controlled the hypertension and got rid of his ED.

Option 4: Taking a Drug "Holiday"

Note: Drug-free "holidays" are limited to non-life-threatening conditions where this option will work without risk to the patient. Discontinuing a beta-blocker, blood pressure medication, or diabetes drug can cause serious complications. If you take daily medication to manage conditions like hypertension, cardiovascular disorders, or asthma, don't stop. Your most important job is to successfully treat your primary condition. Not taking a drug—even for a day—in order to achieve an erection is extremely dangerous to your health.

Many of my patients who take antidepressant medications have adapted their sex lives to their use—a three-day medicine-free schedule, for example. Kirk was one such person. The thirty-eight-year-old, who had been under treatment for depression for several years, was overjoyed when he found that the regimen worked for him. "This is a terrific compromise," he told me. "My depression is under control with Zoloft and I can enjoy my weekends. Life is good."

I began using this alternative therapy after I read an intriguing 1995 study in the *American Journal of Psychiatry* by Dr. Anthony Rothschild. In his small sampling, Dr. Rothschild instructed the men to discontinue their SSRI drugs after their Thursday morning dose and restart them, at the same dosage, the following Sunday afternoon. After four weekends, Rothschild noted that there were no significant changes in the depression levels of those men who took the mini–drug vacations. However, there was definite improvement in both sexual functioning and satisfaction levels. According to him, antidepressant drug holidays worked best with men taking Paxil and Zoloft.

Option 5: Constantly Being Alert to Newer Treatment Options

Every year, new drugs with greater ability to overcome disease are introduced. With their use, the way that physicians treat an ailment can change. This was the case with migraine headache, a condition that has been treated with beta-blockers, calcium channel blockers, and antidepressants. While certainly effective on migraine, these drugs are associated with ED. Patrick, who had suffered from excruciating headaches since he was twenty-eight, responded well to Procardia, a calcium channel blocker. Sometimes a low dose of Elavil, an antidepressant, was added.

But despite the relief they gave him, Patrick wasn't happy with this drug regimen because it gave him another headache: erection problems. The recent introduction of Imitrex (sumatriptan), a very effective drug that could stop a migraine headache within a matter of minutes, became an option. This drug is used on an as-needed basis; as soon as symptoms begin the patient takes it.

While Patrick still experiences migraines from time to time, to his great relief the Imitrex knocked out the pain within half an hour. No longer dependent on prophylactic treatment, he had a spontaneous return of his erections and hasn't had a problem since.

Option 6: Timing Sexual Activity

Making use of chronotherapeutics—the practice of timing drug delivery to coincide with the body's rhythms so that effects are highest when needed and lowest when not—is a relatively new idea that makes a lot of sense. By programming a medication dose to the body's twenty-four-hour physiological cycle, also known as circadian rhythm, a person can receive medicine when his body can use it to full advantage. With chronotherapy, an ailment can be better managed, sexual side effects can be minimized, and the possibility of lowering dosages exists.

Researchers know that every bodily function, from hormone levels and blood pressure to sexual performance, varies regularly—and predictably—during the twenty-four-hour period. They also are aware that the antisexual side effects of many drugs are often diminished or nonexistent just before it's time for the next dose.

They have seen that drugs act differently, depending on when they are taken and what is happening to the body at that time. For instance, hypertension levels are highest upon awakening. Awareness of this fact has led to the development of a new controlled-release medication called Covera-HS. This combination hypertension and angina pectoris drug contains verapamil hydrochloride, a commonly prescribed medication that has been reformulated to be released at a specific time. The pill is taken at night, but the medicine is not released until four to five hours later. Since the drug provides the greatest help when it is needed most—in the early morning hours—and lesser amounts during the day, the user has a much larger window of opportunity for sexual activity.

I saw this happen with Tyrone, a forty-three-year-old with high blood pressure whose medication was causing ED. When I suggested that he try Covera, I explained that everyone's sexual timetable and function have their own particular rhythm, but that for men, the best time to take advantage of the cycle is early in the morning. At that time, body temperature is rising while cortisol, the hormone that speeds up the release of energy-producing glucose in the blood, is also gradually increasing, peaking upon awakening. Testosterone levels usually surge between four and five o'clock in the morning. Add to this the fact that any other medication is at its lowest ebb before the morning's dose, and that a man is likely to be at the least-stressed point of his day, and you have a formula for peak sexual power.

Tyrone's response was extremely positive. The Covera worked for him and, as he told me, "I was always a morning man; I just never knew why. Now I'm back on my regular cycle."

But if none of these options work for you, there is a new fallback position. The new erection pills can be taken half an hour before you want them to work. With their incredible ability to override sexually inhibiting side effects of so many medications, you have the where-withal to reintroduce spontaneity into your love life.

More Good News About Viagra and Vasomax

The man currently taking any number of medicines—either prescription or over-the-counter—that give him ED is now able to counteract the negative condition without compromising his health. Research bears this out. Dr. Harin Padma-Nathan, director of the Male Clinic in Santa Monica and an associate professor of urology at the University of Southern California, has had extensive clinical experience with both Vasomax and Viagra. His findings, which relate to men taking antihypertensive medication, are extremely positive. He says, "ED will be much less of an issue for men taking hypertensive drugs."

One of the pivotal trials with Vasomax suggests it overrides the ED-inducing effects of antihypertensive medications. In the study, men were allowed to continue with their current prescription. When the testing was over, researchers analyzed the data to see if hypertensive medications, a single class of drugs which cause more ED than any other, were still inhibiting sexual function. The results were conclusive: Vasomax was also equally effective in restoring erectile function, whether a man was taking antihypertensive medication or none at all. Vasomax was also effective in men who had mild to moderate dysfunction, whether they were taking medications for other conditions or not.

Dr. David Ferguson, clinical director for the American trials with Vasomax, is even more optimistic about the ability of the drug to override ED-related side effects of medications. He states, "You can improve function while still getting all the benefits of the other medications you are currently taking. In my experience, Vasomax seems to be compatible with all other drugs."

This has been borne out in cases with my own patients. Gary's story is an excellent illustration of the restorative powers of the oral intervention in the face of a serious disease. When he first came to see me, the forty-one-year-old advertising executive had dangerously high blood pressure. My immediate concern was that, left unchecked, his hypertension could lead to a heart attack or stroke. Naturally unnerved by the news, Gary was shattered when I informed him that hypertensive medication very often causes ED. His response was a very common one: "Forget it! Why can't you give me something that will let me live the way I want to? Do you really expect me to give up my sex life?"

I explained to Gary that he had a life-threatening condition but that we could try several different drugs to see which one least affected his sex life. Finally capitulating, he said he would try a prescription. However, when he came back several weeks later, his blood pressure readings were unchanged. Suspecting that he had cut—or even eliminated—his medication, I confronted Gary, asking him if that was the case.

"Okay, you caught me," he confessed. "I did try the medication— but as soon as I did, I couldn't get hard anymore. Look, it's my life and I make the decisions about it, okay?"

I told Gary that in my view it wasn't okay, and that compromising his health in such a dangerous fashion was something I could not condone. Having reached a stalemate, Gary left my office, telling me he wasn't planning to start taking his medicine again.

But later, after I became involved in the Vasomax trials, one of the first men I thought of was Gary. When I called him, he admitted that he was worried about his health. He still had erections, but he'd experienced some problems over the past year, he said. And then there was the untreated hypertension. He said he felt that he was a time bomb that could explode at any moment.

Once I told him about the anti-ED medication, he was game to try it. One week after taking the most effective antihypertensive medication for his condition, Gary felt his ED had worsened. Then he enrolled in the Vasomax trials. The anti-ED drug worked. Ecstatic, he reported to me that he never felt better. "I'm so relieved. I have my health—and my sex life—intact."

ED medication is also effective for men on cholesterol-lowering drugs. When Michael, fifty-seven, came back to my office after his ultra-fast CT test, the special five-minute heart exam confirmed the presence of plaque in his coronary arteries. This was not surprising; he had a family history of heart disease coupled with his own high cholesterol levels.

I prescribed Lopid (gemfibrozil) to lower his cholesterol and triglyceride (fatlike substances) levels in his blood and reduce the risk of a heart attack. Lopid seems to work by raising the level of high-density lipoprotein (HDL) cholesterol, which counteracts the effects of the low-density lipoprotein (LDL) cholesterol, the type that increases the chance of having a heart attack. I informed Michael that the drug would probably work well for him—but that it might also cause erection problems. Knowing the danger he was in, Michael agreed to start medication at once.

At his next visit, I was satisfied to see that his cholesterol levels had dropped to an acceptable level—210 mg—and that his triglycerides had plummeted as well. But Michael's reaction to the good news was one of indifference. "Sure, the results are great," he sighed. "But I can't have sex—so, I still don't feel so good."

I explained that now that his life-threatening condition was under control, we could address the medication's side effect. As part of the Vasomax trials, he tried the pill.

A month later, Michael's wife, Louise, called me. "I just want to tell you myself how grateful we are. Knowing that Michael is healthy is such a relief. Knowing that we can be together the way we want is a gift."

For those men battling depression with medication, there is hope as well. For Richard, a thirty-five-year-old lifelong depressive, taking Prozac was, in his words, "like watching a dark curtain lift and seeing the sun again." With his life and outlook much improved, he began dating and was several months into a loving relationship when he came to see me. "I'm perplexed," he began. "Sometimes I can't get an erection and other times I'm really hard—but I don't come."

Under treatment with a therapist, Richard rejected the idea of switching to another SSRI medication to see if his erection problems would disappear. He felt that the mental stability he had achieved with Prozac was too precious to jeopardize. Instead, he wanted to know if the erection pills could work for him.

I informed Richard that information on the ability of Vasomax to overcome the sexual-inhibiting effects of the SSRIs was limited. So far, few of the men participating in the trials were on antidepressants. The same was true with the Viagra studies. I went on to say, however, that the anecdotal evidence I had seen with Vasomax was positive and worth pursuing. In Richard's case, the results he achieved with Vasomax were consistent with that of other patients: the SSRIs did not hamper the workings of the pills, and his erectile problems disappeared.

PICKING THE RIGHT ANTI-ED DRUG

There are specific instances where one erection pill will be preferable over the other; sometimes one drug is incompatible with a medication currently being used. Consider the story of Jake, a fifty-three-year-old carpenter with coronary artery disease.

For five years, Jake had been taking long-lasting sublingual nitro-glycerin daily. He knew he would be taking the pills for the rest of his life. But, overall, he was in fine health. His job kept him physically active, he was careful about his diet, and he avoided as much stress as he could. But he did have one very significant blight in his life—his life-saving medication was contributing to the gradual loss of firm erections. When he heard about a Viagra trial being conducted at a local clinic, he immediately volunteered.

Unfortunately, he wasn't a suitable candidate. The study coordinator informed him that since he was using a nitrate medication and couldn't switch to another medicine, he had to be barred from the study. Jake fit the sole exclusionary criterion for Viagra: anyone taking a nitrate-based drug cannot use Viagra. In combination with nitrates, the ED pill can produce a host of serious adverse effects in some individuals.

Luckily, a nurse told him that other oral medications were being developed and tested, and eventually he ended up in my office as part of the Vasomax trials. He was enormously relieved to find out that Vasomax has no known negative interaction with drugs, including the one he was taking.

Jake had a very positive response to Vasomax. He told me, "Having a heart condition doesn't limit me in any way. I feel—and act—ten years younger. This is the best thing that could have happened to me."

The fact that Jake took good care of himself helped him a lot. And the same holds true for all men. That's why I developed my virility-enhancement program to make you look, feel, *and* perform better.

The Virility-Enhancement Program

SEXUAL WELL-BEING has always been an integral part of the overall health profile of my patients. It makes a lot of sense: if the body is sound, it is likely that sexual performance will be, too. And the reverse is true as well: if a man's sexual health is compromised, then his body may be in jeopardy. Your first line of penile health defense is determined by three things: supplements, diet, and exercise. All three go a long way toward helping you avoid ED.

The lifestyle recommendations in my virility-enhancement program have more than one application. Not only will they help prevent and, in some cases, treat, ED, they will actually make you feel and look better. And they will not only improve your sexual function, they may also save your life.

Research has shown that optimal sexual health depends on certain lifestyle choices. All affect the body, the flow of blood, and delivery of

173

a pivotal element: oxygen. Although there are several major physical causes of ED, each one has an impact on oxygen flow. They are hypertension, high cholesterol, diabetes, stress, smoking, alcohol consumption, and lack of exercise. Without sufficient oxygen supply to the penis, an erection won't happen. That's because decreased oxygenation of penile tissue can cause progressive fibrosis—a permanent thickening and stiffening of tissue—of the gland. With more fibrous tissue than muscle tissue in the penis, this can cause the penis to actually shrink in size. The crucial oxygen pipeline can be severely limited or blocked by all of the conditions listed above—and all of them can be controlled, improved, or even eliminated through lifestyle changes.

STARTING THE PROGRAM

Health is a dynamic state that can, and will, break down from time to time. Most men experience their first case of ED in middle age, but I personally believe those occurrences can be avoided. That's because —physical and psychological causes notwithstanding—ED is often a disease of lifestyle choices. But even if you know that your ED has a physiological or psychological basis, following the program will still give you added benefits, too. It has been designed to improve your body and mind, and enhance the effects of the oral medications.

The thing to remember is this: habits don't change overnight. The last thing you need is to feel pressured to follow each and every suggestion at once. That's why I've divided the program into three easy-to-follow sections. Each one has advice on supplements, dietary adjustments, and exercise.

The most important thing to do is start. And once you have started and see how well you feel, my best guess is that you will make the recommendations a lasting part of your life.

THE VIRILITY SUPPLEMENTS

Based on extensive research by scientists, as well as my own experience, I have put together a list of seven supplements which can improve penile health. These substances have other wide-ranging effects. Not only can they decrease the risk of ED, they also offer increased protection against cardiovascular diseases such as atherosclerosis.

The seven are vitamin E, vitamin C, Pycnogenol, ginkgo biloba, coenzyme Q (also called Co-Q-10), ginseng, and saw palmetto. You may already be taking one or two of them. If so, see my recommendations to ensure that you are taking a high enough dosage to make an impact on your health. Keep in mind that you can try any or all of these supplements. But as is always the case with new remedies, consult with your doctor before you decide which to take, and in what dosage. Five out of the seven substances listed have powerful antioxidant effects (ginseng and saw palmetto have other properties). Utilizing them to your best advantage can help to ward off—or significantly diminish—the effect of one of the body's great enemies: free radicals.

The Free Radical Connection

Unstable oxygen molecules made daily as a normal by-product of the body's need for energy, free radicals are highly reactive biochemical entities that cause molecular damage to cells. If not stopped, they can disrupt the cell's ability to protect itself. Free radicals are also thought to interact with some fats in the diet, making them clog arteries. Additionally, free radical damage is now being linked to hypertension, stroke, Alzheimer's disease, leukemia, Parkinson's disease, and congestive heart failure.

As we age, the cumulative effects of this endless process begin to take their toll. Study after study has shown that free radicals increase the risk of all cancers, including that of the prostate. Free radicals also oxidize LDL (low-density lipoprotein) cholesterol on artery walls, producing a build-up of deadly plaque. If no intervention is made, the endothelial lining of the arteries is damaged. It is this impaired endothelial function that is believed to precede hardening of the arteries, which is the leading cause of heart attack.

Unstopped, free radicals have the limitless potential to harm every part of the body, including the arteries of the penis. However, there is an arsenal readily available that can stop free radical damage. Antioxidants can halt the injury that free radical molecules have wrought, and then repair cellular damage.

The Antioxidant Effect

Recent research from the University of Maryland Medical Center shows how antioxidants work. After being fed one high-fat (50 grams of fat) breakfast, the blood vessel function of twenty healthy hospital employees between the ages of twenty and fifty-four was found to be impaired for as long as four hours. Blood flow had been significantly restricted in the process.

On another day, the test subjects were given twenty times the recommended vitamin doses—they took 800 international units (IU) of E and 1,000 mg of C—prior to eating the same fat-laden meal. This time, the dangerous adverse effects caused by triglyceride-heavy lipoproteins were avoided. The megadose of antioxidants allowed blood to flow smoothly. That smooth blood flow is crucial for good penile health. A simple way to get it—and keep it—is by taking vitamins E and C. Although this was a relatively small study, further research with larger groups may one day prove that it will be beneficial to take the C and E combo just before eating any fat-rich meal.

The Vitamin Effect

Long regarded as the super-defender against free radicals, vitamin E is also thought to help prevent cataracts and even postpone the effects of aging. Currently, there is growing evidence that taking vitamin E in larger doses helps to reduce the risk of heart disease, thereby enhancing penile health in the process.

A recent study of fifty thousand men aged forty to seventy-five found a 39 percent decrease in heart disease risk in those who took at least 100 IU of vitamin E daily. This showed that the substance works to prevent build-up of fatty deposits (plaque) on arterial walls. The same deposits can decrease blood flow to the penis.

Another study, from the University of Texas Southwestern Medical Center in Dallas, divided forty-eight men into six random groups. They were given either a placebo or vitamin E capsules in dosages of 60, 200, 400, 800, and 1,200 IU daily for eight weeks. Blood cholesterol levels were checked before and after the study. Those men who took 400 IU had substantially less oxidation of LDLs—and therefore less likelihood of it sticking to artery walls—than that of any other group.

Studies also show that it is necessary to use supplements in order to get the full benefit of vitamin E, since it's impossible to get adequate quantities from food alone. The RDA is currently 10 mg for men and 8 mg for women—enough to prevent a deficiency, but hardly sufficient to provide full antioxidant protection. Most of my patients who adhere to low-fat, heart-healthy diets never take in enough of the supplement through diet alone. That's because it's found primarily in high-fat foods like nuts, seeds, vegetable oils, and mayonnaise.

The best way to ensure that you're getting enough E daily for penile protection is with a supplement of at least 400 IU (one milligram equals 0.91 IU). But since high doses of the vitamin may interfere with the clotting ability of the blood, check with your physician first if you are taking blood-thinning medication.

A powerful antioxidant that not only prevents damage on a cellular level, vitamin C can also reverse free radical injury. Researchers have long noted the critical role that this substance plays in the prevention of atherosclerosis, once again helping both the heart and the penis. It does so by reducing both cholesterol and fat levels and increasing the permeability, as well as the strength of, all capillaries, the smallest blood vessels in the body.

In addition, research points to a much lower death rate among men who take vitamin C supplements compared to those who took in adequate dietary amounts but no additional supplementation. One study, at the University of California at Los Angeles, observed the correlation between vitamin C intake and death rates of more than eleven thousand people. As a group, the more vitamin C the men consumed, the fewer deaths they suffered—particularly from heart disease. Another large study at UCLA demonstrated that men who took 300 to 400 mg of vitamin C daily had 15 percent fewer deaths from heart conditions, and lived six years longer than those who didn't.

It's very important for you to consider adding vitamin C supplements to your diet. The current RDA is 60 milligrams, and while it may be justified for disease prevention, it is far from optimal for a healthy life. This was proved in a study from the National Institutes of Health, which delved into the varying dosages to determine which was the most effective. The men taking part in the research were first fed a vitamin C–deficient diet. Then they were given it sequentially, in six specific dosages: 30, 60, 200, 400, 1,000, and 2,500 milligrams daily. The results showed that:

- On 30 milligrams the subjects were irritable and fatigued due to vitamin insufficiency.
- On 200 milligrams blood plasma levels were almost totally saturated with vitamin C.
- At 1,000 and 2,500 milligrams the blood plasma was completely

saturated. But at the higher dose, less vitamin C was absorbed from the intestines and more was eliminated in the urine. Also, the urine contained oxalate and urate, two breakdown products of vitamin C that contribute to the formation of kidney stones.

The NIH researchers now believe that an intake of up to 1,000 milligrams a day of vitamin C is safe (and doesn't cause diarrhea), but that dosages above 400 milligrams have "no evident value." But while food is the best source of this vitamin—citrus fruits are superior suppliers, and most other fruits and vegetables contain it—most Americans don't eat enough every day to get the amount they need.

For optimal antioxidant power, I recommend a supplement of at least 200 milligrams of vitamin C daily. When taking this supplement, it's best if you divide your dose in two, taking half in the morning and the other half in the evening. Since the body eliminates vitamin C in the urine in about twelve hours, taking both doses will ensure steady antioxidant protection throughout the day and night.

The Pycnogenol Effect

Another antioxidant, Pycnogenol (pronounced pick-nah-geh-nol) is a patented formulation of nutrient-packed bioflavonoids extracted from the bark of French pine trees. It offers protection to the endothelial cells which line the heart and blood vessels from free radical damage. Flavonoids—vitamin-like compounds naturally found in fruits (especially citrus), vegetables, seeds, nuts, grains, soybeans, cocoa, tea, and wine—help thwart a host of health ravagers, including viruses, cancer, toxic substances, and heart disease.

Water-soluble, Pycnogenol is readily absorbed in the body and performs a particularly remarkable function by prolonging the quantity of vitamin C in the body. Recent research at the University of California at Berkeley has shown that Pycnogenol can have a positive effect on nitric oxide regulation as well. It's nitric oxide that is so critical for the dilation of penile blood vessels at the time of erection.

In addition to aiding the body in neutralizing free radicals, Pycnogenol also decreases blood pressure by inhibiting the formation of angiotensin, a substance in the blood that constricts vessels. Animal studies with Pycnogenol in Hungary have reported a pronounced decrease in both systolic and diastolic blood pressures. And new research is beginning to show that it may assist in lowering blood pressure without ED-producing side effects common to many antihypertensive drugs.

To receive maximum benefits, I strongly recommend Pycnogenol as part of your preventive antioxidant program. For my patients, I prescribe a two-phase schedule: the first part is the saturation phase, the second is the maintenance phase. To begin, the saturation dose schedule is followed for ten days. During that time, Pycnogenol is taken twice daily with meals. The most effective dosage is 1.5 milligrams per pound of body weight daily. For example, a person weighing 140 pounds would take 210 milligrams every day. Then, during the maintenance stage, the dosage is halved. This is the amount necessary to ensure continued maximum effectiveness. The new amount is also taken twice a day with meals.

The Ginkgo Biloba Effect

The healing powers of this ancient tree include that of an antioxidant. When taken over a period of weeks, it's thought that compounds in the plants can help to inactivate free radicals. By guarding cell membranes from damage, ginkgo helps to make blood vessel walls more flexible and keeps red blood cells pliable, allowing them to squeeze through capillaries without getting stuck. This, of course, makes it easier for blood and oxygen to reach the tissues of the penis.

Studies performed over the last fifteen years reveal that the ginkgo may also be useful in improving circulation and preventing cardiovascular disease. In the last decade, hundreds of scientific papers have been published which detail animal and human experiments with the pulverized leaves of the ginkgo tree. All extol the plant's ability to increase and maintain blood supply.

I recommend one 40 milligram capsule of ginkgo biloba three times a day. Ginkgo biloba is sold in health food stores in concentrated tablet and capsule form. Give this mighty plant time to work. Because it can't repair cells that are already damaged, it may take several months before you begin to notice its effects. At that point, it will be offering protection against further damage and blood flow should be enhanced.

The Coenzyme Q Effect

A mighty antioxidant with the capacity to help prevent and combat heart disease—and therefore protect the vessels of the penis as well—coenzyme Q (Co-Q-10) is actually present in every cell of the human body. Critical to the conversion of food to energy, it is found more abundantly in some tissue cells than in others. Concentrations of the enzyme are particularly high in the heart, researchers believe, because that organ requires an enormous amount of energy to pump blood throughout the body.

First isolated in this country over forty years ago, the workings of Co-Q-10 are still not fully understood. Animal studies have shown that, by stabilizing cell membranes and keeping them from being destroyed, Co-Q-10 acts as an effective antioxidant that prevents free radicals from attacking and damaging cells.

Various research has revealed that as we age, we lose significant amounts of this enzyme in the heart muscle. In some elderly patients, the levels are as much as 75 percent lower than those of healthy patients. In fact, these diminished levels may be a strong indicator of impending death from heart disease. In one Swedish study, ninety-four hospital patients aged fifty years and older who had died within the prior six months had considerably lower Co-Q-10 than the surviving patients.

Co-Q-10 can also have a dramatic impact on elevated blood pressure. In a study conducted by cardiologist Peter Langsjoen, along with researchers at the University of Texas at Austin, 109 patients with hypertension were administered 225 milligrams of Co-Q-10 every day. After a few months, this quantity significantly lowered the blood pressure of more than half of the test subjects, enabling many to stop taking between one and three blood-pressure drugs.

The patients who showed improvement rallied within four months of daily use. Their systolic (upper number reading) pressure was down, from an average of 159 to 147, as was their diastolic (lower number reading) pressure, from an average of 94 to 85. With the Co-Q-10 supplementation, more than forty of them were able to stop taking one or more of their hypertension medications. Another twenty began using the enzyme alone to manage their conditions.

Remember: If you are currently using antihypertensive medication, do not stop taking it. Consult with your physician about starting supplementation of Co-Q-10 in addition to your medicine.

Co-Q-10 is found in small quantities in seafood, eggs, and in all fruits and vegetables. The average person consumes approximately five milligrams of Co-Q-10 daily. Many experts believe that this amount is much too low to meet the needs of the body—especially after the age of fifty. As we age, Co-Q-10 levels begin to drop; by the time we reach middle age, many of us have barely 20 percent of the amount we had in our twenties. This steep drop-off may be due to free radical activity in the mitochondria, the area in the cells where nutrients are converted to fuel for the body's use.

For men in their forties and fifties I recommend daily supplementation of at least 30 milligrams of Co-Q-10. A more accurate dosage recommendation is based on your body weight: 2 milligrams of Co-Q-10 for each kilogram (2.2 pounds) body weight. If you already have heart disease, or risk factors for it, I suggest you take higher dosages after consulting with your physician. Co-Q-10 is available in health food stores and many pharmacies. I find that the softgel, mixed with oil, is more easily absorbed than the dry tablets.

The Ginseng Effect

As I mentioned in Chapter 2, ginseng has already been shown to have an amazing ability to enhance erections. This herb contains many gensenosides, also called panaxosides, which are biologically active compounds thought to be responsible for its physiologic activity. If you have access to an Asian market, buy whole ginseng roots or "tails," which are pieces trimmed off from the main root. The natural product is expensive, selling for as much as $20 to $30 an ounce, depending on availability. The roots and tails can be chopped, and the pieces steeped in hot water, to make a herbal tea.

How much or how often ginseng should be taken depends on personal need. For men who are thirty-five to fifty-five years old and in good health, small quantities—about one eighth of an ounce of prepared or whole root—may be taken regularly as a tonic. For older men, this dosage can be doubled to one fourth of an ounce taken daily.

A much easier solution is to buy commercially prepared ginseng tonics, powders, and capsules; health food stores and pharmacies stock them. Be sure to check labels for gensenoside or panaxoside content. Price is another indicator of quality; look for higher-priced products manufactured by a reputable company. To get maximum results, follow the label directions.

The Saw Palmetto Effect

A fan palm tree with razor-sharp branches that can be found all over Florida, the saw palmetto is filled with olive-sized berries. The extract of these berries is believed to be a sexual stimulant and a remedy for enlarged prostate glands.

It is the latter application that is particularly interesting. Benign prostatic hyperplasia, or BPH, is a common enlargement of the prostate gland. Very prevalent in men past forty, its exact cause is not fully known. While it is not cancerous—nor does it lead to the disease—a man can have both BPH and prostate cancer simultaneously. And although BPH doesn't affect sexual performance directly, its urinary symptoms can get in the way of sexual activity.

Situated in the front of the rectum and just below the bladder, the prostate completely surrounds the top portion of the urethra, the channel through which both urine and semen pass from the body. A reproductive organ the size of a walnut, the prostate's major function is to produce part of the fluid portion of semen. During orgasm, muscles in the prostate quickly contract, pushing the prostate fluid through special ducts into the urethra, where it mixes with other fluids that help carry sperm out through the tip of the penis.

While the prostate itself plays no role in the urinary system, disorders of the organ often cause urinary problems due to the gland's close proximity to the bladder and urethra. Enlargement of the prostate, due either to BPH or cancer, will often constrict the urethra where it runs through the prostate, contributing to bladder-relieving problems.

All symptoms of BPH are linked to urination. As the prostate enlarges, the flow of urine through the urethra is obstructed. Frequent urination, a difficulty starting the action, a weak stream, and dribbling at the end of urination are typical symptoms. Until recently, surgery was the only option. It has now fallen out of favor for several reasons. For one, it often failed to provide relief. For another, it often led to chronic incontinence. Cases of TURP (transurethral resection of the prostate) surgery could lead to an increased risk of death from cardiovascular disease. On top of all that, it is estimated that as many as 15 percent of men go on to develop ED following surgery.

Now, however, there are prescription drugs that will effectively shrink the prostate or relax the muscle tissue that constricts the urethra. Unfortunately, the drugs designed to control BPH often bring about ED or a loss of libido in many men. Finasteride (Proscar) is one such medication.

Today, many doctors are recommending the use of saw palmetto extract instead of prescription drugs to treat BPH. If you are one of the 50 percent of men over the age of fifty who have developed troublesome symptoms of BPH, talk to your physician about trying saw palmetto. A recent small study of fifty men, conducted at the University of Chicago School of Medicine, found that half taking the extract experienced a 50 percent improvement in urinary symptom problems. While it is not yet known just how saw palmetto works, it does seem to make the urine stream freer-flowing as well as relieve other typical BPH symptoms. And, perhaps most significantly of all, it accomplishes this without any ED-inducing side effects.

If BPH is a concern, consult with your doctor. After ruling out the possibility of prostate cancer with a simple office examination and a blood test that measures the level of prostate-specific antigen (PSA), *I often recommend that saw palmetto be tried. The typical dose is 160 milligrams taken twice daily, a regimen that is continued for up to eight weeks.* If a definite benefit is experienced, then the regimen is continued. If, however, there is no change in urinary condition, then I will try a prescription drug approach to the problem. Typically, I prescribe an alpha-adrenergic blocker such as terazosin (Hytrin) or the newer tamsulosis (Flomax). If the drugs don't work, surgery may be recommended.

If you have a family history of BPH or prostate cancer but have not yet experienced any symptoms, saw palmetto can be a great health aid. Once you reach your forties, consider taking 80 mg of the extract daily. It can enhance the health of your prostate, considerably reducing or even eliminating the chance of developing BPH.

Finally, there is another prescription for BPH, one that does not require medication of any kind. For mild BPH cases, sex at least once a week seems to significantly reduce prostate swelling and eliminate some of the troubling symptoms in the process. Many men find that meeting this minimum, or increasing the frequency of sex to three or more times a week, goes a long way toward reducing symptoms—with no adverse side effects.

And even for men with no BPH problems, frequent sex is a practice that should be seriously considered. Basically, the old cliché about "use it or lose it" is true, at least in this case. A regularly occurring erection supplies oxygen to the blood vessels and tissues of the penis. Maintaining this vital oxygenation reduces the chances of developing erection problems in the future.

THE VIRILITY-ENHANCEMENT DIET

Supplementation is an important part of maintaining and enhancing virility. But, it can't—and shouldn't—be considered a substitute for the right diet that will contribute to your overall health. Even if you adhere to a beneficial diet, you should also be aware of specific foods that will make you feel, look, and perform better.

We all know that a fat-heavy diet is not beneficial. As a general rule, a balanced, low-fat diet with at least five servings of fruits and vegetables daily will do you a world of good. Focusing more meals around carbohydrates (pasta, rice, and beans), with meat as a side dish, is a sound way to eat.

But there is more to consider. You may not be aware of the way that certain foods can lessen the chance of developing ED. All of the foods I am recommending are readily available and you may be eating them already, but perhaps not in the quantities you need. They are: soy, fish, olive oil, flaxseed, and tea. You don't have to ingest massive quantities of them; all you have to do is add them to your diet. Here's why.

The Soy Connection

Soy reduces LDL cholesterol levels while at the same time raising HDL cholesterol readings. A 1995 analysis of thirty-eight human studies that appeared in the *New England Journal of Medicine* found that eating 1.6 ounces a day of soy lowered LDL cholesterol by 13 percent, with almost a 10 percent reduction in triglycerides. Simultaneously, HDL cholesterol rose 2 percent. Dr. James W. Anderson of the University of Kentucky, who authored the report, believes that soy can help cut heart disease risk in this country by 25 percent or more. And that, of course, means that the incidence of ED can be lowered as well.

Researchers have speculated that the high soy intake among the Chinese and Japanese is related to their corresponding low levels of heart disease. Other studies also suggest that soy removes LDL from the bloodstream, delivering it to the liver where it is broken down for excretion. The mechanism for this may be through the actions of substances known as phytoestrogens, a type of plant hormone akin to human estrogen. The result is artery protection from plaque build-up and protection from cancer.

A legume no bigger than a pea, soy is available in many varieties, including tofu (soy bean curd), and soy burgers, flour, milk, and tamari, a sauce. A high-protein, low-fat nutrient that can be substituted for meat, soy should be added to your diet. Just a few ounces a day can improve your health.

The Fish Connection

The concept is very simple: eating fish at least once a week will lower your cholesterol, enhance overall vascularity, and improve erectile health in the process. New studies on the effects of fish eating support the idea that polyunsaturated fatty acids are responsible for this. The omega-3 fatty acids, found primarily in the oils of the fish, lower blood triglyceride levels. The omega-3s seem to make blood less likely to coagulate, which, in turn, makes it less likely to clot. They accomplish this by raising the levels of prostacyclin in the blood, thereby making the arterial walls relax. At the same time, they lower the levels of thromboxane, another chemical messenger which is responsible for the constriction of blood vessels.

One study of 1,300 men showed that those who consumed at least eight to nine ounces of fish weekly (and that was mostly canned tuna) had an incredible 40 percent lower risk of a fatal heart attack than those men who ate little or no fish.

To get the fullest benefits of all fish has to offer, I suggest that you eat it two or three times a week. Fatty species, such as herring, cod, mackerel, salmon, and sardines, contain greater quantities of omega-3s than do leaner varieties. But if the idea of eating that extra piece of fish each week is just not appealing to you, there are other ways to get the omega-3s you need. Flaxseed may be the source that will work for you.

The Flaxseed/Olive Oil Connection

Although flaxseed has been best known as a source of linseed oil, this ancient food which contains both soluble and insoluble fiber is also the richest known vegetable source of omega-3s. A food with incredible heart-protecting properties, flaxseed contains the highest levels of alpha-linolenic acid, a variety of omega-3 fat. Flaxseed oil is another option. Its omega-3s promote the formation of prostaglandins, the hormonelike substances that help to relax capillaries, decrease cholesterol levels, and lower blood pressure.

If you decide to use the seeds, sprinkle a few tablespoons on your cereal, mix them into yogurt, and, if you wish, grind them and add the powder to food. Use the oil as you would any salad dressing. You should be aware that this highly polyunsaturated oil has a shelf life of less than a month and that exposure to heat, sunlight, and air can turn it rancid. It should not be used for cooking. However you use flaxseed or its oil in your diet, just make sure you do so a few times a week in order to get your optimal dose of omega-3s.

Another heart-healthy ingredient, olive oil has been found to be especially helpful in transporting LDL cholesterol out of the body while at the same time guarding HDL cholesterol levels. It is the HDL which protects the heart. This has been observed in coronary disease studies of Italians and Greeks in their native countries. While these people consume about the same amount of daily fat as do Americans, their choice—three tablespoons of olive oil a day—has shown to be very beneficial to their health. (In this country, Americans average three tablespoons of olive oil a month.)

My recommendation is to cut out any butter and margarine you may be using and substitute the best olive oil you can buy instead. Your body will thank you for it.

The Tea Connection

Tea has a lot more to offer besides a caffeine jolt. A recent study that appeared in the *Annals of the Archives of Internal Medicine* reported on 522 Dutch men who drank five cups of black tea—the kind most Americans drink—daily for fifteen years. They had a 74 percent lower risk of stroke than that of a control group. The researchers pointed to the vitamin-rich flavonoids in tea as a possible reason. These particular flavonoids make blood cells less prone to clotting—in about 80 percent of stroke cases arteries to the brain are blocked by clots. And, of course, flavonoids also have a strong antioxidant action.

Black tea isn't the only variety to offer health benefits; green tea also has health properties. In a study of 1,300 men over the age of forty published in 1996 in the *British Medical Journal,* it was found that those who drank significant amounts of green tea—in this case ten cups a day—tended to have lowered LDL cholesterol levels. When compared to non–tea drinkers, these men also had an increased proportion of HDL cholesterol.

Give your body a health boost. Two cups a day of black or green tea will keep your arteries clearer, your blood flowing better, and your erectile capabilities enhanced.

Two to Avoid: Alcohol and Tobacco

Adding all of these foods to your diet will help your penile health. There are two substances, however, that will hurt it: alcohol and tobacco. If you consume more than two alcoholic drinks per day consider cutting back. If you don't, you run the very real risk of giving yourself ED, or worsening an existing condition.

Steady drinking can inhibit both erection and orgasm. It does so by affecting the production of nitric oxide, which, in turn, makes it difficult for the tissue of the corpora cavernosa to relax enough to allow blood to flow in the penis. If drinking continues over time and alcoholism develops, there is even more damage. The peripheral nervous system is often injured, permanently affecting the ability to have an erection.

Excessive alcohol also has a negative effect on blood pressure levels as well. Estimates suggest that in about 7 percent of those with blood pressures of 150/95 or higher, the elevated hypertension is related to the consumption of three or more alcoholic drinks a day. A bottle of 4.5 percent beer, a 4 ounce glass of 12 percent alcohol wine, and 1.5 ounces of 80 proof spirits are each considered one drink. Studies have shown that a reduction in alcohol intake significantly lowers systolic and diastolic pressures in both hypertensive and normotensive men.

If you do drink, do so in moderation.

Many men who drink also smoke. You probably already know the ill effects of this habit, to which ED is another entry on a long list of health-sapping conditions. Smoking causes blood vessels throughout the body to be clogged. And once blood flow is restricted, the ability to have an erection is impaired. A 1994 study of 4,400 Vietnam veterans found that smokers were more likely to admit to ED than nonsmokers and men who had quit the habit. This translated to a whopping 68 percent higher overall risk of ED for smokers. Even ruling out the associated ED risks such as alcoholism, depression, and the use of a number of medications, the smokers still had 50 percent higher chance of developing ED than the others in the study.

The good news is this: if you give up smoking, erections can return within a few months. Your blood pressure will be lower, your blood flow will be better, your heart and lungs will function better, and you will have given yourself more years to actively enjoy a fulfilling sex life.

Virility Exercises

Active is the operative word here. Keeping your body moving will not only make you look and feel better—it will also improve your sex life and decrease the possibility of developing ED. It's difficult to enjoy a fulfilling sex life without a physically active body. At the most basic level, we know that regular exercise improves overall fitness, and that sexual functioning is an important part of the equation.

We are also aware that regular exercise positively affects brain wave activity, making you feel more energized. Body temperature is also raised, duplicating one of the main reactions associated with sexual arousal. Also, the more you exercise, the more muscular stamina you develop, which translates to the prevention or delay of fatigue during sex.

Physiologically, regular physical activity has an impact on vaso-congestion, raising blood supply to the penis and helping to achieve and maintain an erection. On a hormonal level, exercise raises testosterone levels, leading to increased libido. And it works psychologically as well. As the percentage of body fat begins to drop and you are able to exercise longer, self-image can soar. All these factors can positively alter personal attitudes about sex.

There are several types of activities that you can include in your daily regimen. They will restore and maintain suppleness of movement as well as overall flexibility. All are easy, don't require special equipment, and don't cost anything. *They are: walking, stretching, and resistance exercises.*

Walk Your Way to Good Sex

Walking not only enhances endurance by increasing lung capability, it improves the strength and efficiency of muscles in the abdomen, back, and legs. At the same time, it doesn't put any strain on ankles or knees. For men who are out of shape and/or overweight, walking is the perfect exercise. For one thing, you'll be able to walk a lot farther than you would be able to run. That means you'll be able to burn more calories. In a matter of weeks, daily walking can also decrease blood pressure by about ten points. It does so by improving the body's sympathetic nervous system. And by lowering blood pressure, walking enhances penile health.

Start with an easy stroll—about one to two miles an hour—and gradually work your way up to striding or race walking, which covers about five miles an hour. If you find that you can't fit in a daily walk, go for a shorter one whenever possible. Quantity, not quality, counts here. You don't have to walk nonstop for thirty minutes to get the full advantages. Even short five- and ten-minute intervals throughout the day will yield health dividends.

And don't forget to include your partner in your walks, not only for the companionship, but also to enhance her sexual arousal. Intriguing new research from the University of Washington's Human Sexual Psychophysiology Laboratory in Seattle has found that it's exercise —by increasing heart rate and body temperature, priming a woman to respond to sexual stimulation—and not so much the fabled romantic candlelight dinner that leads to sexual arousal.

Stretch Yourself

To promote flexibility—the ability to use muscles and joints through their full range of motion—you should stretch at least three times a week. Regular stretching also helps to relieve stress, a major contributing factor to ED. When performed in a slow and focused way, stretching can be excellent relaxation therapy as well as a tension easer. Here's the correct way to do it to avoid injury.

Static stretching calls for gradually lengthening through a muscle's full range of movement until resistance—or discomfort—is felt. To maintain flexibility, an optimal session should last from ten to twenty minutes, with each stretch held for at least ten seconds. Then work up to holding each for twenty and then thirty seconds. To increase flexibility, stay in the stretch for one or two minutes.

Tight hamstrings are a major cause of poor back flexibility and back pain, which can lead to a diminished sex life. To relax the hamstrings, do the following two exercises daily. The morning stretch should be performed just after waking up. Sit on the edge of the bed with your feet flat on the floor and your knees at a 90 degree angle.

193

Keeping your knees together, bend forward at the waist, letting your chest touch your knees. Hold the position for ten seconds. Repeat five times. If you need a greater stretch, push your feet out farther from the bed.

The second stretch is the straight-legged hang. To do it, stand with your feet flat on the floor and your knees locked. Bend over from your waist and try to touch your fingers to the floor without straining. Without flexing your knees or bouncing, hold the position for one minute. Remember: if at any time you feel pain stop the stretch.

To fully enhance flexibility, you might want to consider taking yoga or T'ai chi. An ancient Chinese art whose slow-controlled movements can help increase suppleness, strength, body awareness, and balance, T'ai chi is a series of choreographed, dancelike movements. One British study of heart attack victims found that the slow, deliberate motions and breathing patterns of T'ai chi lowered the heart rates of some people.

One of the goals of yoga is to enhance muscular and joint flexibility. A discipline which puts a great emphasis on deep breathing and slow body movements, this Eastern series of exercises helps to increase the range of motion in tendons, muscles, ligaments, and joints. Yoga postures encourage muscles to extend to their full length, something years of slumping over office desks while sitting in poorly designed chairs has sorely inhibited. An added benefit of all the various postures, called asanas, is improved blood circulation.

Here are some very basic yoga stretches that will increase flexibility of the spine and pelvis and ultimately enhance blood flow to the penis. Do them every day. When you perform these exercises remember to breathe in sync with the movement and slow your pace, concentrating on every aspect of each motion.

The first stretches are a modified version of the Sun Salutation (Surya Namaskar), which is a sequence of a dozen positions performed as one continuous movement. To begin, start with the hurdler's stretch

(Figure A). Stand with your left leg bent at the knee, toes pointed

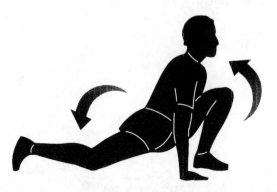

FIGURE A

forward. Stretch your right leg straight out behind you, flexing the foot gently. Let your pelvis slowly drop toward the floor as you bend the knee of the left leg. Hold the stretch for twenty seconds and repeat with the opposite leg. When you're finished, the next four movements should flow one after another. Bring both legs back and get into the classic push-up position (Figure B), with your hands directly beneath

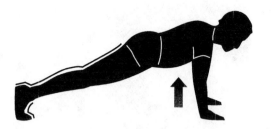

FIGURE B

your shoulders and your knees straight with your hips. Your weight is now supported by your hands and toes.

While taking a long, slow breath, lower your chest, keeping your pelvis up (Figure C). Slowly lower your pelvis to the floor (Figure D),

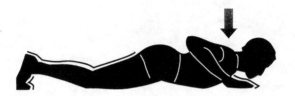

FIGURE C

point your toes, and slowly push up with your arms. Keeping your pelvis on the floor, bend your low back as you gently stretch and look toward the ceiling.

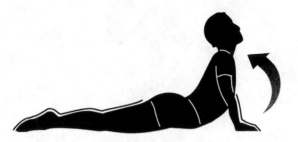

FIGURE D

Now, curl your toes under, raise your pelvis, and get into an inverted V position (Figure E). Keeping your heels flat on the floor, try

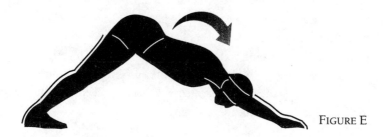

FIGURE E

to touch your forehead to the floor. Take a step forward with either the right or left foot and place it between your hands. You are now back in the original (Figure A) starting position. Repeat this entire sequence of stretches.

The next stretch is for the inner thigh and will help loosen your groin area. Lie on your back and extend your legs up a wall and rest your heels there (Figure F). Make sure the back of your pelvis is

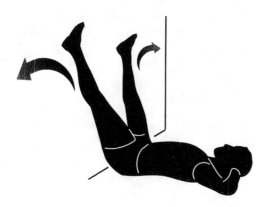

FIGURE F

touching the floor and that your legs, as wide apart as is comfortable for you, aren't too stiff. If they are, move back from the wall. Slowly press the backs of your knees and legs against the wall. Breathe deeply to help release the tension in your legs, letting the full weight of your torso relax downward. Hold this position for one or two minutes. If your knees feel uncomfortable, bring your legs closer together.

The last exercise is a simple groin release, modified from the classic yoga lotus position. This stretch will help to relax your adductors, the five muscles that start at the top of the thigh at the pubic bone and extend along the inner thigh to the inside of the knee. To perform this stretch, sit down on the floor with a straight back and bent knees (Figure G). Place the soles of your feet together and pull the ankles inward so your heels are near your crotch. Resting your elbows on the insides of your knees, lean forward from the waist so that your elbows push your knees toward the floor. Hold the stretch for twenty seconds and repeat three to five times.

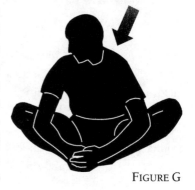

FIGURE G

The Acupuncture Connection

Traditional Chinese medicine attributes acupuncture's healing powers to its ability to restore a normal balance in vital life forces called *qi* (pronounced chee). Qi is believed to move through fourteen major meridians—invisible energy-carrying channels—throughout the body. Each channel is associated with specific organs, and every acupuncture point is considered to have a particular therapeutic benefit. The energy flow can be accessed at many points along the meridians. Some Western researchers have suggested that acupuncture works by stimulating pain-blocking neurochemicals—either endorphins (the powerful substances produced in the brain that deaden pain and alter mood), or painkillers that are generated near the site where the needle is inserted.

Acupuncture has long been used in Asian countries as a way to treat men with ED. In this country, Alfred Peng, M.D., the president of the American College of Acupuncture, has had some success helping men with mild or moderate ED. Dr. Peng, an associate clinical professor of surgical science/pain control at New York University Medical School, believes that, in theory, the technique increases blood flow to the penis. He states, "Acupuncture is excellent for increasing microcirculation in the body. I'd recommend six to seven sessions. If you notice improvement with your sexual function, continue with the acupuncture treatment."

To treat ED, thin stainless steel needles—about the thickness of a human hair—are carefully placed in the lower spine and coccyx, as well as in the groin. They are inserted less than a quarter of an inch below the skin's surface, and usually left in place for fifteen to twenty minutes. Little, if any, discomfort is felt. Some people describe the sensation as a mild tingling.

Acupuncture is performed in every state in this country. An estimated three thousand medical doctors and osteopaths have studied and used acupuncture in their practices. Approximately seven thousand nonphysician practitioners currently use the technique to help control pain and treat addictions, depression, insomnia, and other health problems. You should be aware of the licensing regulations in your state. To find a physician/acupuncturist in your region, contact the American College of Acupuncture at 212-876-9781.

Note: Before trying acupuncture to treat ED or any condition, consult with your doctor. As is the case with other forms of alternative medicine, acupuncture should be used only as an adjunct to regular medical treatment—never as a substitute for it.

Learn How to "Resist"

If muscle fatigue during sex has become an unwanted presence in your life, you need resistance training. This type of exercise will increase overall muscular strength in your arms, abdomen, back, and legs. To measure the current state of your muscles, get down on the floor and see how many push-ups you can do in a minute. A man in his forties should be able to perform at least twenty. A fifty-year-old should be able to manage fifteen. If you can't meet these numbers, start performing this classic exercise daily.

To test your midsection strength, see how many crunches you can perform in a minute. Lying on the floor with knees bent, feet flat on the floor, and arms crisscrossed over your chest, curl up until your shoulders come off the floor. Then return to the starting position. I expect a man in his forties to be able to do anywhere from twenty to forty crunches. A fifty-year-old should be able to accomplish at least fifteen in sixty seconds. If these numbers are high for you, add crunches to your daily regimen.

If you really want to build muscle strength, ten to twelve repetitions with light weights for each muscle group two times a week will be very effective. Get a professional to show you what to do to avoid injury.

Remember: regular aerobic exercise, such as walking briskly, running, or swimming laps for twenty minutes or more several times a week can protect against ED development. However, for all of you men who ride a bicycle there is an ED connection that you should be aware of: prolonged sitting on the traditional narrow riding saddle.

Recent research by Dr. Irwin Goldstein, the internationally recognized ED expert, bears this out. When a man sits on that narrow seat, his entire body weight presses down on the cavernosal artery, the major blood pathway to the penis. Several hours in this position can lead to possible erection problems due to compression of the artery, as well as other blood vessels. According to Dr. Goldstein, it takes only 11 percent of a man's weight to compress the artery when he's sitting on an un-padded racing-style bike saddle.

If you are a regular bike rider and are experiencing numbness in your penis after a ride, you can halt—and reverse—any potential dam-age. One option is the recumbent bike. With its wide chair, all the rider's body weight is supported by the sit bones, the bony protrusions of the pelvis. There are also new saddles available that take all pressure off the cavernosal artery. Some models have a wide hole running down the middle; others have a shorter nose. Both will protect you while you get the benefits of riding.

Taking care of the physical component of your life is vital if you want fulfilling sex, as is understanding the emotional underpinnings of your relationship. There is, however, one more part to the sexual fulfillment puzzle that you must be aware of if you are going to have the best sex of your life.

Reigniting Your Sex Life: Yours and Hers

As YOU HAVE seen throughout this book, a fulfilling sex life requires a lot more than a pill. There are any number of variables and conditions which can affect the attraction, as well as the performance, of two people, with one factor overriding all the rest. Without libido, the desire to bond physically with another person can be greatly diminished—or even lost. A constant presence throughout our lives, libido ebbs and flows as much as the tides. Springing from an intricate network of physiological and psychological components, libido varies from man to man. And, of course, from woman to woman.

Years of living with ED can have a profound and far-reaching effect on the libidos of both men and women. When sex is absent, often the desire to have it again is sacrificed as well. Yet, when sexual function is restored—as it can be with the new oral medications—libido doesn't automatically jump-start in both partners equally, much less simultaneously. For many men, the desire to have sex is a logical extension of being functional again. For women, however, the reality can be very different.

Many women have told me so. Their husbands or companions, ecstatic with the return of their potency, exhibit an intense longing for sex. But often the women don't. It's not, they explained to me, because they don't feel attractive or because they no longer have feelings for their partners. Rather, it's because they have adapted to their situation, integrating the loss of sex into their daily lives. And, they confess, the idea of accessing those dormant feelings can be daunting.

Their reaction is totally understandable. The longer they have lived with men who have ED, the harder it can be for them to tap into their own sexuality. As you read in Chapter 6, there are many ways to heighten intimacy between partners. But where libido is involved, the approach is somewhat different. The best place to start is inside your head.

THE POTENCY OF MEMORY

Where libido—and indeed, one's entire sexual being—is concerned, there is a single organ that supersedes all others: the brain. If you are a man in a long-term relationship, it's likely that you're very aware of your partner's desires. But maybe years of living with ED has made you put them on hold. Now that your problem is under control and you're ready to have sex, think about your partner.

Begin by remembering the person who attracted you. This is the person you fantasized about. Recall those times when you were closest. Consider that she is still there with you, but doesn't have a pill that will help to boost and restore her sexual longing. To help her unleash those sleeping passions, you need to reestablish an emotional connection. Your desire for her must be conveyed in the ways that you remember she likes. These, of course, will vary greatly from couple to couple. But you know yourself—and your partner. It's up to you to go the necessary distance.

Without acknowledging the other person's wants and needs, sex cannot be the totally encompassing event that you hope it will be. Getting to know someone well does take time—and is worth the effort. A person whose longings and pleasures are recognized is going to be a lot more receptive than one whose libido is dismissed or ignored. Not paying attention is an added stress, which can only serve to harm your relationship.

THE STRESS FACTOR

If you thought that stress couldn't tamper with your life any more than it already has, consider this. Stress can dampen sexual arousal. An action that includes the surging of blood, increased heart rate, and erection, arousal depends, to a great extent, on a number of various hormones to spark specific reactions in the body.

But there are other hormones discharged from the adrenergic system—epinephrine and norepinephrine, especially—that can effectively shut down sexual response. Whenever you are under stress, no matter what the source is, these hormones begin to course through your veins, directing blood flow to the heart and major muscles and, therefore, away from the genitals, in both men and women. This results in increased heart rate and blood pressure, two physical factors that can contribute to lowered libido and performance.

GETTING BACK IN SYNC

Synchronizing your sexual longings with those of another person will reward you over and over again. If you or your partner has a sex drive which has slackened off, you owe it to yourselves to find ways to build it up again. This has to be a joint venture; if one person is in the mood for sex and the other couldn't care less, then there obviously is going to be a no-win situation. Finding that mutual connection takes time and thoughtfulness. What might work for you—a porn movie, for instance—could be a big turn-off for her. On the other hand, slow dancing might be your partner's preferred way of building to a sex-filled night, but the idea leaves you cold.

One of the best, and mutually satisfying, ways to reignite libido is to rediscover the pleasures of touching. Dr. Robert Broad suggests that partners need to steer away from focusing on the act of sex itself. "There are other ways to use tactile communication with your partner," he states. "Zero in on touching, one of the most powerful components of human sexuality. Using tactile communication, including kissing, caressing, and petting, just as you did in early courtship, will help you to reexplore sexual sensation and bond you together. They can amp up your sex life because of the tremendous numbers of sensory receptors that are in the skin."

Sexual researchers, therapists, and counselors have found communicating with your partner through increased touching to be one of the most effective means to expand intimacy and add vitality to a sexual relationship. Many couples find that giving each other a massage is a great way to enhance their mutual attraction as well as boost libido.

GET BACK IN TOUCH

The following exercises will allow you to explore the erotic sensation of your skin and that of your partner. Taking the time you need and want, these movements can promote closeness and trust. Done with gentle, caring hands, these massages can lead to sex. But don't regard them as foreplay. Rather, they should be performed to give, and receive, pleasure. And when that happens, the possibilities to go forward are always there. But before you begin, do both of yourselves a big favor. Set aside a generous chunk of private time and make sure that you can't hear a ringing phone.

To begin, wear as little clothing as you are comfortable in. Or, if you choose, nothing at all. Sit on the floor or bed with a pillow between your crossed legs. Have your partner rest her head on the pillow. Then take a small amount of massage, coconut, or safflower oil in your hands and stroke it gently and rhythmically on your partner's forehead. Using both hands, work your way smoothly across her closed eyes, her nose, and down across her cheeks. Feel the texture of the skin under your fingertips, and be aware of the planes and contours of the facial surface.

Never losing touch with her body, softly cup both of your hands around the back of her head and, with a steady motion, gently massage her scalp. Move down to the neck, massaging the underlying muscles which store tension. Then proceed to the shoulders, all the while manipulating your hands on her skin, absorbing the rising heat of her body. Think about how she is responding and how you feel. Does this intimate exercise stir a longing for more touching? If so, proceed to the next step.

If there is anything that a stressed-out person deeply appreciates, it's a back massage. Strong hand movements up and down the back trigger nerve fibers and increase blood flow and circulation by dilating blood vessels. The result is a relaxation response that both of you will enjoy.

To start, have your partner lie on her stomach. Straddle her lower back comfortably. With your palms facing downward, make gentle circles around each shoulder blade. Then, using the knuckles of both hands, stroke her back from the neck down, about two inches away from either side of the spine. Explore the contours of her back with rotating fingers and deep kneading motions. Finish the massage with slow strokes. As one hand, with fingers spread wide, makes its way up the length of her back, the other should descend to the lower part.

As you progress, ask your partner how she feels. Find out if you are applying too much or too little pressure. Ascertain what feels good to her and what she doesn't like. Tell her how touching her body and giving her pleasure affects you. Paying a person this kind of undivided attention can be a big turn-on.

The Neurotransmitter Connection

Keep in mind that everyone's sex drive is different. And although no one is certain why one person has a stronger sex drive than another, neuroscientists are beginning to unravel and better understand the workings of the libido. One thing we do know: when two people click, it has as much to do with chemistry as it does with biology. Among the key factors that influence libido are the neurotransmitters dopamine and serotonin. These brain chemicals send messages to the nerve cells, playing an important role in determining our sex drive.

Now recognized as a crucial ingredient in sexual arousal, dopamine is ultimately responsible for evaluating the many sensory stimuli you encounter in the course of the day. As that information—which is comprised of what you see, hear, smell, taste, and touch—is perceived by your brain, the dopamine system rewards you with heightened sensory states.

Nestled deep in the brain stem, dopamine is the so-called pleasure chemical messenger that makes us feel good. However, the brain is very stingy with dopamine, only releasing it from its cells for brief moments. When the neurochemical is discharged, it plugs keyholes, called receptors, on other cells. Once it has done this, dopamine is picked up by transporters and is stored and conserved for future use. Normally, the release of dopamine is pulsed on and off as needed. But, in some men, the discharge of this brain chemical is less frequent than it is in others. When this happens, the man is said to have a low libido. In other words, he just doesn't seem very interested in having sex.

Serotonin has a different role. A calming neurotransmitter, it has a significant effect on mood, aggression levels, what foods we crave, and how much of them we eat. Too little of this chemical can result in sleep disorders, rage, and food binges. Too much, however, isn't good either —it can have a decidedly negative effect on your sexuality. As we saw in Chapter 8, drugs which promote the release of serotonin can cause a decrease in sexual desire.

THE TESTOSTERONE EFFECT

Scientists also know that libido is linked to the male sex hormone testosterone. Technically an androgen, a type of steroid that acts as a male sex hormone, testosterone provides the masculinizing elements that orchestrate development of muscle tissue, the lowering of the voice during puberty, and overall growth, including that of the penis. It has other consequential applications as well, affecting libido, memory, and lean body mass. Interestingly, at birth, boys have the same testosterone levels as young adult males. They drop quickly, however, and remain low until puberty. At that time they rise, setting in motion the development of masculine characteristics.

Testosterone production continues to climb as men get older, eventually tapering off at around the age of forty. At that point they drop off about 10 percent each decade. By the time a man reaches sixty, his level may be one third what it was between the ages of twenty and forty. In that period of time, his reading ranges from 300 to 1,000 nanograms per deciliter of blood. It's estimated that about one third of men over the age of fifty have lowered testosterone levels, and by the age of sixty-five, more than 60 percent have low testosterone. Despite a lowering of testosterone, the "free" testosterone levels usually remain in the normal and adequate range. It's only a distinct minority of men who require some testosterone supplementation. The hallmark of the testosterone-depleted man is decreased libido.

Nature may have intended testosterone to decline with age. The body may be guarding itself against the enlarging of the prostate gland —which grows in the presence of testosterone—by dropping down normal production of the hormone. Still, the significance of that decline remains unclear. Circulating in a man's bloodstream and acting on his brain to enhance his sexual desire, the hormone may also intensify penile sensation. Testosterone levels rise and fall throughout the day; some researchers think there is an hourly difference. There is even a monthly variation. Typically, testosterone levels are lowest in February and highest in the autumn.

But despite the fact that testosterone has a very pronounced effect on libido, it has little to do with whether or not a man achieves an erection. Even so, some doctors mistakenly link diminished testosterone levels with erectile dysfunction and prescribe testosterone patches or monthly injections for their patients. Raising minimally depressed testosterone levels rarely, if ever, improves erections.

Testosterone replacement is highly controversial, except in cases of men with a condition known as hypogonadism. Men with this ailment have extremely low levels of testosterone—under 300 nanograms per deciliter—due to decreased function of the testes. Their symptoms include lessened libido, mood swings, insomnia, irritability, decreased bone mass, weakness, lethargy, and loss of lean body mass. These men also have decreased erection capability, an overall drop in sex drive, and are at risk for osteoporosis.

A Testosterone Boost

When a man is truly testosterone-deficient, replacement can work wonders. This was the case with a fifty-four-year-old patient named Bill. When he couldn't help but notice the progressive decline of his sex life, he quickly—and wisely—brought it to my attention. A man who enjoyed a regular sex life with Emily, his wife of twenty-three years, Bill was incredulous. "I'm losing my urge to have sex," he said. "I guess it's sort of inevitable at my age—maybe I just don't have all the testosterone I used to."

I told Bill that his assessment was probably right and ran a blood test to support our view. His hormone level measured a low 220 nanograms—any reading under 300 is considered deficient. After checking for evidence of abnormalities that could be contributing to his deficient levels—testicular or prostate cancer, pituitary disease, and cirrhosis of the liver are known offenders—and coming up negative, I recommended that he have an injection of testosterone.

A few days after getting a shot of 200 milligrams, Bill reported back to me; his libido had definitely been stirred. After two more weeks, he received a second shot, and soon afterward, I switched him to prescription transdermal patches. With them, he could easily self-medicate. Each night he placed two patches on his body, on either a thigh, an upper arm, his back, or abdomen. Each 2.5 milligram patch gradually released the hormone through the skin and into the bloodstream. After a month of using the patch, Bill called me again. "I have that old urge back," he told me. "It feels like an old friend has come back for good."

Research at the St. Louis University School of Medicine has found that giving men an injectable form of testosterone for three months increases their sex drive as well as augments muscle strength. And a study conducted in 1995 at the Chicago Medical School found that a low dose of testosterone given regularly for two years seemed to cause no side effects. According to a researcher involved in the study, the men receiving injections felt better, had denser bones, lower cholesterol readings, and a greater sexual appetite than men who weren't getting the supplementation.

But, hypogonadism aside, I don't believe that there is sufficient scientific evidence to warrant testosterone boosting in men with normal levels. If a man is given testosterone supplementation when he really doesn't need it, his pituitary and hypothalamus—which would normally signal testosterone production—slow down or stop. Once the pituitary gland is suppressed, the testicles begin to atrophy and the man becomes sterile. Another side effect is blood thickening, which can lead to a greater risk of stroke. Extra testosterone can also promote prostate cancer.

If you feel that your libido is drooping, you can raise your testosterone levels naturally. Start a strength-training program that works the muscles of the torso and legs. After a few workouts, there will be a short-term surge of testosterone. This natural boost can be maintained by continued exercise and you will have the added benefit of a stronger body and finer muscle tone. Another factor to consider when evaluating yourself is stress. When pressure starts to rise, testosterone levels begin to fall.

SELF-AWARENESS IS THE KEY

You now know the physical, psychological, and emotional elements that constitute a fulfilling sex life. You've seen how diet, supplements, and exercise can make a huge difference in your performance and enjoyment. And, most importantly, you have available to you new oral medications, simple and easy to take with virtually no side effects, that can help overcome erectile dysfunction. But the rest is up to you. And being aware of yourself—and your partner—as sexual beings is the most important element of a fulfilling sex life. Yet if you do experience problems—for whatever reason—the new world of sexual medicine can help. The Virility Solution is yours.

Acknowledgments

In our book we have spoken about the pioneering work done by Dr. Adrian Zorgniotti and Dr. Irwin Goldstein as well as other leading urologists and researchers in the field of sexual medicine. We would like to pay tribute to these dedicated people for their invaluable contributions and thank them for their discoveries now and in the future. We feel privileged to have learned from these experts.

The preparation of this book went far beyond our dual efforts and required the assistance of many. We would like to thank them especially, because without their support this project would not have been possible. Our agents, Herb and Nancy Katz, are surely the best, most caring, meticulous, and enthusiastic agents any author could want. These publishing visionaries served as our editorial advisors and guiding lights, working tirelessly from the initial planning stages of the book straight through the final review process. Fred Hills, our longtime editor and friend, was an enthusiastic ally and insightful supporter of the project right from the start. Thanks as well to Carolyn Reidy, who believed in the importance of our message. We would be remiss if we did not acknowledge the fine assistance and editing prowess of Burton Beals and Hilary Black, who improved the book. We would also like to extend our heartfelt thanks to Susan Suffes for her thoughtful attention, invaluable contributions, and many late nights and lost weekends spent shaping and reviewing the manuscript. Her unfailing assistance helped make this a better book as we raced to meet an ever-challenging deadline.

Our special thanks go to Dr. Robert Broad for his valuable contributions in the development of the psychological component of the manuscript that became Chapter 7. Our gratitude is also extended to the many doctors who took time from their busy schedules to offer helpful comments: Dr. David Ferguson, Dr. William Greenfield, Dr. Eli Lizza, Dr. Ian Osterloh, Dr. Harin Padma-Nathan, Dr. Alfred Peng, Dr. Raymond Rosen, and Dr. Pierre Wicker. Tim McInerney, David Brinkley, Andy McCormick, and Kate Robins also provided important contacts and helped steer us along our path. We would also like to acknowledge Dr. Lamm's patients, as well as those referred by Dr. Michael Brodherson, Dr. Jeffrey Glasser, and Dr. Steven Kallet. Many of these men were involved in the Vasomax medication trials and graciously agreed to be interviewed about their struggles with ED. We learned so much from them and their partners. The publication of this book has been inspired by their desire to achieve the Virility Solution.

Steven Lamm, M.D., and Gerald Secor Couzens
New York

Index

INDEX

INDEX

hypertension, 31, 41, 48, 51, 82, 99, 113,
    132, 148, 149, 150, 164, 166, 168,
    190
hypogonadism, 209–10
hypothalamus, 30, 211
hypothyroidism, 82

Ignarro, Louis, 59–60
insecurity, sexual, 124–26
insurance, 37
International Index of Erectile Function
    (IIEF), 90–92, 100
    questionnaire, 92–100
*International Journal of Impotency
    Research,* 29
Iphiclus, 25

jimsonweed (*Datura stramonium*), 28

Langsjoen, Peter, 182
libido, 20, 30, 53, 76, 91, 95–96, 99,
    106, 134, 148, 153, 156, 185, 192,
    202–11
Lizza, Eli, 38, 41–42
Louis XVI, King of France, 27
Lue, Tom, 65, 66–67, 130

Male Clinic, 167
mandrake plant, 26
Marie Antoinette, Queen of France, 27
Massachusetts Male Aging Study
    (MMAS), 149–50
massage, 205–7
masturbation, 76, 95, 109, 134
mechanical devices, 26, 33
    see also vacuum erection therapy
Medicare, 37
medical research, 10, 55–58
medications:
    antacids, 157
    antidepressants, 29, 150, 153, 164–65
    antihistamines, 150, 156–57
    antihypertensive, 167, 182
    beta-blockers, 151, 164, 165
    calcium channel blockers, 151, 165
    cardiovascular, 150–53, 164
    as cause of ED, 48–49, 54, 58, 147–72
    clinical trials of, *see* clinical trials
    diuretics, 151, 163, 164

ED chart of, 160–61
gastrointestinal, 150, 157–58, 159–60
oral erection, *see* oral erection
    medication
psychiatric, 150, 153–56
tranquilizers, 150, 153
vasodilator, 149
see also specific medications
Melampus, 25
Melman, Arnold, 130
meloid beetle, 30
men:
    self-esteem of, 88, 105, 108, 125, 129,
        145
    sexuality and, 24, 102–3, 105, 129
    treatment resisted by, 145–46
migraines, 165–66
Mount Sinai Hospital, 140
multiple sclerosis, 47
MUSE, 37–38

National Institutes of Health, 133, 178–
    179
Native Americans, 28
nerve disorders, 46–47, 58, 65, 81
neurochemicals, 199
neurotransmitters, 30, 35, 59, 207–8
New England Journal of Medicine, 187
New York Times, 148
New York University Medical School,
    199
nitric oxide, 45, 58–60, 61, 180, 190
nitroglycerin, 171
norepinephrine, 30, 204
Norvasc, 148

obesity, 47, 50, 51
olive oil, 187, 188–89
omega-3 fatty acids, 188–89
oral erection medications, 10, 11, 18
    effects of, on relationships, 129–46
    ethical concerns and, 132–37
    and men, 116–19, 134–35, 138, 167,
        202
    and women, 135–36, 138–43
    see also Vasomax; Viagra
orgasm, 30, 91, 98, 154, 184, 190
Osbon, Geddings, 33
Osbon Medical Systems, 33

217

INDEX

About the Authors

Steven Lamm, M.D., is an internist and Clinical Assistant Professor of Medicine at the New York University School of Medicine. He received his undergraduate training at Columbia University, and his medical degree and clinical training at New York University School of Medicine. A panel physician for the New York State Athletic Commission, Dr. Lamm is a regular guest on New York network television news programs, offering his analyses and comments on a wide variety of health- and medical-related topics, and is frequently quoted in national magazines. He is the author of two renowned medical books, *Younger at Last* and *Thinner at Last*. He lives in New York City with his wife and children.

Gerald Secor Couzens is the former syndicated fitness columnist for *New York Newsday*. He writes about fitness and health issues for various publications. He lives in New York City with his wife and children.